MW00477339

BRAVE NOW

B

N

**Rise Through Struggle and
Unlock Your Greatest Self**

RADHA RUPARELL

Brave Now: Rise Through Struggle and Unlock Your Greatest Self – 1st edition

ISBN 978-1-7366094-1-5

Published by: Woodacres House

Contents

Download Your Free
Action Guide Now

As a gift to my readers to help you get the most out of this book, I encourage you to download a FREE action guide with daily micro-practices to use alongside this book.

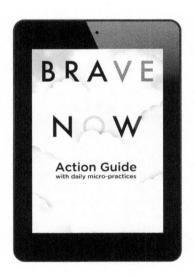

Go to www.bravenowbook.com/bonus
to download today!

Foreword

On April 5, 2020, I started to feel tired, more tired than I would usually feel in the middle of the day. Two days later, I found myself trying to catch my breath on a conference call. It was then I first suspected that I had been hit with this new virus that everyone was talking about, COVID-19. Being in my late thirties, I thought I would recover quickly. I had no idea then the long journey ahead of me. Nine months later, I am still very much in the fight as I write this.

This disease is like nothing I have ever experienced in my life. I started the year as a healthy, single, young professional working in Manhattan, living an active life, traveling often for work and pleasure, and enjoying the company of good friends on weekends.

Then I contracted this virus and suddenly found myself bedridden, unable to work, and suffering from a full-body assault on my heart, brain, stomach, and other organs.

After 16 days of quarantine fighting this virus alone in my New York apartment, I could no longer hold it all in. During a bout of insomnia, I opened my computer and started writing. I wrote about the debilitating effects of this virus on my mind and body, and the lessons I was learning as I battled it. The next morning, I uploaded this short piece: "What No One Tells You About Having COVID-19" to the publishing platform Medium, and shared it with family and friends.[1] So little was known about COVID-19 at the time that I was simply hoping to encourage my loved ones to take it seriously and stay safe.

Within two weeks, more than 20,000 people had read my article. I was overwhelmed at the outpouring I received. Hundreds of loved ones and strangers reached out with words of support and many of them shared with me their own stories of loss and hardship. Several people encouraged me to keep writing, and so I did. Whenever I could muster a little energy between bouts of pain and fatigue, I would write a few words. That is how this book came to be.

This is a story about the battle I faced, but more importantly, about the life lessons I discovered along the way. While battling this illness, I felt haunted, scared for my life, in pain, confused, anxious, angry, alone, worried that I was losing my mind, and terrified of others getting sick. I also had the most profoundly beautiful experiences of self-discovery, connection, gratitude, creativity and love.

When I first shared my story with others, several people told me that I was brave. I couldn't even comprehend that at that time as the virus had hit me so severely that it was a struggle just to get out of bed in those early days.

Over the coming months, however, I had time to reflect on the question: What does it mean to be brave? While I discovered many lessons through my own journey, I was also deeply inspired by the resilience of so many others who battled this virus themselves; the frontline healthcare workers who put themselves at risk every day; the droves of resilient teachers who found ways to keep kids safe and learning under dire circumstances; the working parents who juggled extra responsibilities at home and work; and so many other brave souls who valiantly took on an unprecedented year with all their might.

I know for sure that being brave does not mean the absence of fear. I will admit that I encountered fear many times over the past months. What I have discovered is that perhaps being brave means: taking on each day newly even in the face of fear; treating yourself and others with compassion even when it's hard; embracing adversity as a source of wisdom and connection; and being vulnerable enough to let the world experience the real you, perfectly imperfect, just as you are. Being brave is not an innate characteristic reserved for a select few. At any moment, any one of us can choose to be brave.

From a young age, we are conditioned to put up shields and hide ourselves from others, yet it's precisely the things we hide that make us human. When we open up and allow both our struggles and our strengths to be a welcome part of who we are, we can begin to connect more deeply with the people and world around us, and also with ourselves; and if we embrace this wild ride of life, with all its ups and downs, with a little curiosity and generosity, we might just discover the key to unlocking our greatest selves.

Let's stop hiding and embrace all of who we are. How sad it would be to reach the end of our lives never having shown up as our full, powerful selves. If this year has taught me anything, it's that we may not have tomorrow. So be brave, I say. Be brave now!

Warmly,

Radha Ruparell (December 5, 2020)

Introduction: Turning Point

Turning point

Sometimes it takes a catastrophic event to wake us up. We get diagnosed with an illness, end a relationship, lose a loved one, get fired from a job, or are faced with some other event that completely disrupts life as we know it. One minute, we're doing well, the next, we're in the middle of a crisis. Turning points can be terrifying. Yet one thing is for certain: we will all encounter these moments in our lives. The ultimate question is, how are we going to face them?

Here's what I have discovered. While turning points can be disorienting, you always have a choice about how to respond. You can either let these moments knock you down, or you can discover your inner strength and rise up stronger than you started.

Cultivating this inner strength is like building any new skill. It requires learning how to do it, and then a lot of practice and perseverance.

This book is for you if you have ever faced hardship and uncertainty and want to equip yourself to deal with these situations more powerfully. Or if you're simply feeling stuck in life and are yearning to get unstuck. I use the story of a turning point in my life—my battle with COVID-19—to share how you can deal with any turning point in your life. You cannot always change your circumstances, but you can develop the inner capacities to deal with any circumstance that life throws at you.

This book is also for those who see this moment in time as a collective turning point for humanity. It's almost as if this virus has lifted a veil on what needs to transform, both in the world around us and the world inside us. In the world around us, millions of lives have been turned upside down by a global pandemic that restricted our ability to move freely, gather, earn a living, go to school, feel safe, and care for loved ones, among many other things. In our inner worlds—our hearts, minds and souls—we are facing similar struggles as we confront fear, anxiety, uncertainty and loss at heightened levels.

Disruption can be terrifying and daunting. Yet it can also be a source of creativity and new beginnings. Without disruption, we are not capable of knowing how much we can grow. Disruptive moments might be exactly what we need to transform ourselves, and the world around us.

My hope is that whatever your own turning point is, this book might offer you some inspiration to: stand tall in the face of adversity; rediscover beauty and connection in everyday moments; and unleash your full, powerful self in the world!

Paralyzed with fear

In April 2020, at the age of 39, I was struck with COVID-19. Prior to that, I was a healthy, single, young professional working in Manhattan, living my best life.

In just a few days, life as I knew it collapsed into complete disarray. Physically, I experienced sensations that I couldn't have imagined a week earlier. In my first week, I felt like I was losing control of my body. I had deep bouts of fatigue where I felt like someone had drugged me with a bottle of sleeping pills, and for hours a day, I couldn't even muster the energy to get out of bed. Headaches were so bad that

I thought the pressure might cause my head to explode. Night fevers brought haunting hallucinations. I would fall asleep for a couple of hours, often to be jolted awake gasping for air.

By the second week, the symptoms had progressed to a point where I was truly scared for my life. On Day 8, I wondered if I was having a heart attack. I had shooting pains all night, and my left upper chest felt constricted. The doctors told me that under normal circumstances, I should be hospitalized, but since New York was the epicenter of the pandemic, hospitals were in danger of being overrun, protective equipment was scarce, and beds were being reserved for those in direst need. So I, along with thousands of others, was asked to manage symptoms from home, have telehealth consultations, and take on heavy drug regimens that would normally be monitored under supervision at a hospital. By the end of that week, I had also lost my will to eat and had shed seven pounds.

In the third week, the battle became more mental. Unlike a typical illness where there is a steady progression, this disease was constantly morphing, as if it had a mind of its own. Just when I thought I had it beat, it would come back in another form. One day I was dealing with the worst headache of my life. The next day, I had an elevated heart rate, chest pains, and shortness of breath. It was like a disorienting, never-ending series of curveballs.

This virus was also unusual because it came in waves throughout the day. For fleeting moments, like when I was writing this, I was lucid, could form words—I felt almost normal. And then in a matter of minutes, I would find myself bedridden, completely unable to move, and in a brain fog where I couldn't focus my attention for even a few seconds. I consider myself mentally tough, but as I battled this, many times I felt like I was losing my mind!

By week four, I was forced to confront extremely difficult questions. Would this ever end? And if it did, would I even be myself again? I asked myself this question over and over again one night after facing an especially deep brain fog and numbness in my face that left me in a complete stupor. No matter how hard I tried to focus, I couldn't access certain parts of my brain. Stringing together a complete sentence suddenly felt out of reach. *Surely, it's temporary*, I thought at first. But deep down, my biggest fear was *What if it's not?* What if I'd had a mini-stroke and would never be the same? What if this virus caused permanent damage to my brain? The body pains were similarly unnerving. While I have experienced pain many times in my life, this felt different. At moments, I felt as though the lifeforce was being sucked out of my body, as if my body were giving up for good.

One night, I was sitting in bed, lucid and responding to a text message, and in just a matter of seconds, my vision went blurry and my body became so limp that I thought to myself, *This is it.* I tried to get out of bed, but as I did, I collapsed to the ground. I fumbled to pick up my phone that had fallen with me. I was so disoriented that I could barely pick it up, but after a couple of shaky attempts, I finally managed to dial 911. Luckily, the paramedics arrived quickly and I recovered from that incident, but when I returned home from the hospital, I mustered up the courage to do something I had been dreading for a while but knew had to be done. I opened up my computer, not a month before my 40th birthday, and wrote up my will.

Navigating uncertainty

After a month of going to bed at night wondering if I would make it to see the next day, I finally started to have real hope that I would survive this. The symptoms continued to cycle in waves, but it was reassuring when the chest pains got a bit milder than the week before, or when fatigue kept me down for only a few hours rather than the whole day. The challenge was that, even though I was making progress, it still felt slow as a snail, and it definitely did not follow a straight path.

The unpredictable nature of this illness has been one of the most traumatizing things I have ever faced in my life. I am usually good with uncertainty, but this illness really pushed me to the edge. It was volatile on so many levels: how it cycled through my body with different symptoms each day; how it presented so differently across different patients; and how poorly understood this virus was among the medical community, especially at its outset.

Imagine facing a week of chest pains, then they subside, and then BAM! Out of nowhere, two days later they come back in full force. It's mentally exhausting to think you're free of something only to find yourself back at square one. But that's exactly how this virus operates. And it's not just one symptom, it's all of them: chest pains, shortness of breath, pounding headaches, nausea, deep fatigue, body aches, tingling, numbness, joint pains, stomach issues, elevated heart rate, dizziness, brain fog, and insomnia, to name just a few. They come. They disappear for a while. And then they come back again a few days later, sometimes with a vengeance. You never get the feeling that you're ever truly winning. And you're always anxious in anticipation of what's going to hit next.

On top of all this, since this illness was so new, those who were not suffering from it could not always truly relate to it. Understandably so. We're familiar with illnesses like the common cold that have a fixed set of symptoms and a straight-line trajectory. Unfortunately, this virus plays by its own rules.

Even the doctors who treated me did not fully comprehend the erratic nature of the disease. What made it even more challenging for them was that the symptoms presented quite differently in different patients. Some patients came in with a cough, low oxygen, and pneumonia. Others presented with nervous system sensations, including a loss of smell and taste or tingling in the body. One patient would recover in fourteen days while another would struggle for several months. An elderly person might suffer because their immune system was not strong enough while a young person might suffer because their immune system was too strong and had overreacted to the virus. There is no "normal" for this disease, which made diagnosis and treatment even more of a crapshoot.

Finally, since I was one of the earlier cases in the US, little was known about the virus and its effects when I first became ill. With doctors working around the clock to manage the overwhelming surge of new patients, few had enough time to pause and reflect on what was really going on. When I was in my first week of this, most doctors were treating COVID-19 as if it were primarily a respiratory disease. Since my oxygen levels were relatively normal at that time, the healthcare providers I worked with didn't take me very seriously. However, by my fourth week of the disease, the medical community had started to realize that this virus could affect every single organ in the body. It could attack the respiratory system, gastrointestinal system, or nervous system. It could ravage the heart, lungs, brain, liver, and many other organs. At this point, the doctors started acknowledging the symptoms that they had filtered out before, yet so much still remains unknown about this novel virus.

The uncertainty of this all was extremely distressing. I had friends in the medical field tell me in despair that they just didn't know enough about this disease yet and were at a loss for what to do with my case; that they were throwing the "kitchen sink" at sick patients but not sure what was really working or not; that drugs given to patients in the early weeks of the virus's onset were later banned once mortality data started coming in. It was an honest take on what was going on, but frankly, not very reassuring.

In my second month of this illness, I saw every type of doctor possible, and they were all learning alongside me. The neurologist found a brain lesion in my frontal lobe. The cardiologist gave me a heart monitor to wear 24 hours a day because my resting heart rate was 20-30 beats a minute higher than it should have been and very erratic. The gastroenterologist tried to help me with the nausea that made me feel like I was living on a ship in a stormy sea, among many other stomach issues that plagued me for weeks. The infectious disease doctor shared that it was likely that my body's own immune system was now attacking me, and that COVID-19 could trigger dormant viruses and possibly spark a long-term autoimmune condition.

While each doctor helped in their own small way, none of them really knew exactly how this virus was operating or what it would take to cure me. The virus was still very much a mystery, and I could tell that these interactions were anxiety-provoking for the doctors, given how little they knew. On top of that, they were putting themselves at personal risk every time they faced an infected patient. It was terrifying for me too, knowing that these doctors were still just taking shots in the dark. As my symptoms progressed, I was acutely aware that what was at stake was not just a few weeks lost to a fleeting seasonal illness. What was at stake was my life.

Embracing a new reality

In the months that followed, I discovered an online community of people who continued to suffer symptoms way beyond fourteen days. In the early months of the pandemic, this extended version of COVID-19 was mostly neglected by the medical community and the media, but at a certain point, there were too many of us to ignore. We created a name for ourselves, "long-haulers," to illuminate the sad fact that even months after the virus's initial onset, we were all still facing a slew of disturbing symptoms. While my symptoms got a little less severe week after week, I would quickly relapse if I over-exerted myself physically or mentally, and that was true for many other long-haulers.

Luckily, I have a job where I can work from home, so after a couple of months of being completely debilitated, I started slowly returning back to work. While no day was exactly the same, the following describes a day that felt quite typical at this point in my fight:

I'm jolted awake after three hours of sleep to find my heart racing at 160 bpm (the rate that it would be at if I was running at full speed). I start my day by taking seven different medicines that the doctor has prescribed me, including two self-injections.

I work for a couple of hours and then a wave of fatigue and pain hits me. I feel the urge to lie down, but I can't do that because laying down triggers a massive pain in my left ear like a drill boring through my head. I take a walk outside, hoping it will relieve the pain or at least distract me from it for a little bit.

The doctors have requested a lot of tests, so it's quite typical for me to walk over to the local lab for tests. On this day, however, a nurse comes to my home for a blood draw. I'm terrified of needles, and so the kind nurse tries to distract me with small talk while I sit on a stool on my kitchen counter. By the fifteenth and final vial, I can feel myself getting faint and motion to the nurse that I need help getting to the couch where I promptly pass out. When I come to, the nurse waits a couple of minutes before jetting off to her next visit. I slowly get up and force-feed myself lunch.

In the afternoon, I sit down to work again and find that I just can't focus due to brain fog. I try for a bit and get very frustrated. Finally, I give up and go for a walk again in my local park. Watching the runners whiz by me reminds me of a time when I had stamina. For now, I can barely walk to the park and back without getting short of breath. I come home and take my evening meds and injections and prepare for another night of restless sleep. This is my new reality.

Wondering "Will it End"?

Normally a news junkie, I usually love to keep up with what's going on in the world. However, after a couple of months of this illness, I made a conscious choice to stay away from anything that would put me in a negative state of mind, and that included the news. Every once in a while, though, I couldn't help myself and would scan the headlines.

One Sunday, as I was reading the newspaper, I caught wind of a hypothesis in the medical community that some COVID-19 survivors would end up with lifelong conditions. That morning, I sat in the park and cried for the first time in a long time. While the first few weeks of the virus had been terrifying because I feared for my life, this new prospect of having a lasting chronic illness felt even more daunting.

Prior to this virus, I was healthy in mind and body. I meditated, surfed, played tennis, and walked around Manhattan with a New Yorker's hurried gait. I lived a fast-paced life. And then COVID-19 hit me. Now, nine months later, while I have regained much of my strength, I wonder if I will ever return to full health again.

Facing the turning point

So how did I confront this turning point in my life? Mostly, I found myself drawing on the many life lessons that I had accumulated over the years through my personal and professional journeys. At one point, I had an epiphany: perhaps every single thing I had experienced up until this point in life was simply a training ground for this very moment.

In my day job, I run a Leadership Accelerator at Teach For All, a global network of organizations in more than 50 countries that are developing collective leadership to ensure all children have the opportunity to fulfill their potential. Through this work, I have the good fortune of working with incredible leaders from around the world who are reimagining education in their own local contexts. A core belief behind this Accelerator is that if we want to transform systems around us, we first must be willing to transform ourselves, or as the saying inspired by Mahatma Gandhi goes, "Be the change you wish to see in the world." As I have supported incredible leaders around the world to grow their inner leadership, I too have been on a journey to grow my own leadership. The tools and practices I have been exposed to in this field of leadership development served me well during my battle with this virus.

My whole life, I have also been an avid reader, and stories of others have inspired me to dream bigger, battle adversity, and cultivate my curiosity. I now want to contribute back in the hope that sharing my experience can help even one person in the way that others' stories have lifted me up over the years. In that spirit, I am sharing with you a set of lessons that helped me through my battle with COVID-19, and that will continue to be guiding lights in my life much beyond this experience.

I hope that these lessons can provide some inspiration for you too as you face turning points in your life.

PART I

BUILD RESILIENCE

1

Lean and be seen

Allow yourself to lean

The single most important thing that helped me through my COVID-19 battle was having a strong support network. In the days after this virus first hit me, I had barely any strength. My phone felt like it weighed one hundred pounds, and I would get short of breath speaking a few words. So initially, I reached out to a doctor friend and to my sister for support but no one else. But soon, a work colleague of mine, who I would not have expected to be one of my core pillars of support, started reaching out to me every day. Her encouraging text messages offered me so much comfort and helped me get through the difficult nights. And then, I began reaching out to others. I found comfort in a friend who brought me humor, another who helped me get groceries, and an online COVID-19 support group that let me see that I was not alone in this.

I used to think that reaching out for help implied weakness, that strong people don't complain and can tough it out. Now I believe the opposite: that admitting you can't do it on your own is not weak at all. What I have learned is that, especially in times of collective trauma, having a broad support network matters, and that we should ask for the help we need. Admittedly, I felt quite raw and vulnerable at times, but with nothing left to lose, I shared my deepest fears and thoughts with others in ways that I had never done before. In doing so, I allowed many people to support me and was humbled by the incredible warmth I experienced as I let my fate become intertwined with theirs.

Allow yourself to be seen

What is it that stops us from being vulnerable? I can tell you that I felt very exposed at times sharing myself so openly. When you let someone into your inner world and they see all of you—your fears, your frustrations, your weaknesses, as well as your love, your appreciation, your dreams, and your strength—it is a profoundly intimate experience.

I think what stops us from revealing ourselves fully is that we make the false assumption that we are alone in these emotions. Of course, if we are being completely rational, we know that other people, too, feel love, joy, sadness, fear, anger, shame and guilt, just like us. Somehow, though, we all walk around the world with masks on, protecting ourselves from being fully seen or from the risk of being judged.

But what would happen if we just removed those masks for a moment?

I gave removing my mask a shot on Day 16 of my illness when I wrote that short article about my COVID-19 experience and shared it with my entire personal and professional network. For some people, this might not seem unusual at all, but for someone like me who rarely posts on social media and guards my private thoughts very closely, this felt like an extremely vulnerable act.

What I discovered in removing my mask was that on the other side lay connection—a deep human connection with others so beautiful and profound that it completely stirred my soul, leaving me grateful rather than resentful that I had endured this harrowing journey.

In sharing my story, I connected with: a 60-year-old stranger who discovered a "renewed sense of hope and optimism" around her own circumstances; another stranger who shared that he now feels more confident in how he might battle this virus should he get it; a former work colleague who shared with me that she too had suffered from a debilitating disease; a great aunt in London who hosted a virtual puja (prayer) service in my name; co-workers around the world who sent me pictures of the outdoors (forests, gardens, waterfronts!) in their hometowns to lift me up beyond my four walls; and hundreds of other people who shared their love for me and my family, or confided in me about their own traumatic life experiences.

How ironic that I was sitting in quarantine in a New York apartment by myself for a month, and yet I felt more deeply connected to humanity than ever before. In these times, we are all wearing physical masks. But what if we removed the invisible masks that we've been wearing since long before this virus began? What is it that you are hiding from others? And what might be possible if we all started opening up and unveiled what was really underneath our masks?

Bring your whole self

Right before I fell ill, the magnitude of what we were facing globally had just started to sink in. As the pandemic unfolded across the world, I first experienced the feeling of angst and fear at my workplace, Teach For All, as I interacted with colleagues all around the world who were being affected by the pandemic in different ways.

In the early days of the pandemic, we hosted video calls where colleagues from around the world would get together. At the beginning of these calls, we would take a few minutes in small groups to check in with one another personally. In these moments, I learned that some colleagues had family members infected with COVID-19. Others were struggling with working from home while parenting young children. Many were facing the daunting challenge of reimagining education in their countries in the wake of indefinite school closures. These precious spaces to pause and be with one another were a chance to bear witness to each other's raw realities. In these moments, we also discovered our deep interconnectedness.

I'm hopeful that in this new era, we will begin to shed the idea that we need to fit into our professional environments with outward personas that are different from who we are at home. What if, instead, we removed our armor and engaged with one another more authentically all the time? Yes, it might feel intimidating to take that leap, especially in workplaces where our personal and professional sides have been siloed for much too long. But the truth is, we are whole human beings, and trying to fit into some fake mold of how we "should be" is exhausting. It disconnects us from ourselves and from one another when what we are really craving is belonging and connection. Our workplaces are where many of us spend the majority of our days, so what a tragedy it would be to spend the bulk of this time in hiding.

I have learned that it only takes one person to inject vulnerability into a space for that space to become real rather than superficial.

Perhaps that person could be you.

2

Let go and be with what's so

Be with what's so

On Day 14 of being sick, I finally broke down. In a text exchange with a good friend, I admitted, "I have never been more scared in my life." For two weeks, I had been resisting my fear. My fear of dying. My fear of losing loved ones to this illness. But finally, when I was able to just "be with" that fear and say it out loud, suddenly it wasn't as terrifying anymore.

So often, we don't even create space in our lives to acknowledge our deepest thoughts and emotions.

Instead, we keep ourselves busy and find ways to distract ourselves through work, social media, television, eating, drinking, making jokes and other distractions. But when we force these feelings to stay beneath the surface without acknowledging them, they gnaw away at us in ways we don't even realize.

One day, early in my illness, I was feeling completely overwhelmed. I had been up all night with a fever and night sweats, and I desperately wanted to take a shower, but I was so weak in the morning that the journey from my bed to the bathroom felt like a marathon. I finally made it out of my bed and staggered the few short steps to the bathroom. As I opened the bathroom door, I remember staring ahead at the shower and then suddenly realizing I didn't have the energy to stand for even a moment longer.

Overcome with emotion, I sat right down on the bathroom floor and I let everything out—frustration, exhaustion, and anger. I had been suppressing these emotions for too long. But in that moment, sitting there on the bathroom floor, I just allowed myself to feel. It was quite cathartic, actually! Sometimes the simple act of allowing these emotions to be there, rather than pretending they don't exist, is all we need to loosen the grip they have on us.

Inspired by a poem by the Persian scholar Rumi, I have learned to treat emotions such as fear, anger, sadness and overwhelm as visitors in my house. When I notice them, I try not to suppress them. I allow them to enter for a moment, embrace the wisdom they are offering me, and then eventually let them go. I'll admit that this is not always easy, but we can develop this capacity with practice.

Mostly, I have discovered that while we cannot stop our thoughts and feelings from arising, we do have a choice about how we relate to them. If we're overcome by our emotions in certain moments, there is nothing wrong with that. Oftentimes our feelings are a source of wisdom. For example, on days when I was feeling overwhelmed, it was usually my body's way of telling me that I needed more rest.

The important thing is that we grow our capacity to notice our thoughts and emotions without being completely beholden to them. We don't have to suppress them, but we don't have to let them consume us forever, either. We can simply let them visit for a while and see what we discover.

The Guest House

This being human is a guest house.
Every morning a new arrival.
A joy, a depression, a meanness,
some momentary awareness comes
As an unexpected visitor.
Welcome and entertain them all!
Even if they're a crowd of sorrows,
who violently sweep your house
empty of its furniture,
still treat each guest honorably.
He may be clearing you out
for some new delight.
The dark thought, the shame, the malice,
meet them at the door laughing and invite them in.
Be grateful for whoever comes,
because each has been sent
as a guide from beyond.

— Jalaluddin Rumi, translation by Coleman Barks
(The Essential Rumi)[2]

Let go of resistance

There is a saying that "what we resist, persists," and I find that this really holds true. In times of uncertainty especially, it's not our circumstances that destroy us; it's our resistance to them. In this rapidly changing world, we have to accept that we can never fully control our circumstances. And that's hard because so many of us are wired to want total control! But the more we try to control things, the greater resistance we face, and this chips away at the very power we were trying to cling on to in the first place.

As one example, when I first got sick, I kept thinking to myself, I just need a couple more days and then I'll be back at work. I would let my team know that I'd be out of commission for a few days but that I'd be back on Monday. But as Sunday approached, I would start feeling dread in my stomach because I knew deep down that I was not ready for re-entry yet. And each week, as I reneged on my original promise to my co-workers, I felt massive pangs of guilt and disappointment.

Finally, after a couple of weeks going back and forth like this, I accepted the truth. That week, I did not tell my team I would return on Monday. Instead, I shared with them that I would return when I healed and I wasn't sure when that would be. In letting go and just allowing myself to be with the uncertainty of it all, I finally found some freedom. In particular, I found freedom from the shame that had been crippling me when I felt like I needed to "get somewhere" on a timeline that I now realize was completely untenable.

This lesson in letting go of resistance came alive for me again a couple weeks later when I started facing neurological symptoms. So little was known about the virus when I first fell ill that I was eager to read as much as I could about the latest medical findings to see if there was anything that might shine light on my condition.

But when I tried to read, I struggled with brain fog. I would find myself staring at a news article reading the same sentence over and over again with no memory of the words I had just taken in. Or as I attempted to watch the news on TV, even with 100% of my energy focused on the task, I could not absorb a word the news anchor was saying. These experiences were beyond frustrating. I'm usually a pretty calm person, but in these moments, I wanted to scream at the top of my lungs in pure frustration.

At first, I tried to power through this brain fog, but the more I tried to focus, the worse things got. I started developing debilitating headaches every time I tried to concentrate too hard. Finally, one day, after going through this ordeal over and over again for many days, I realized I had no choice but to listen to my body. That's when I gave up resisting.

To give up resistance, I had to learn to let go. I had to let go of activities like reading and television that my brain could not handle at that moment. What came next, though, was a pleasant surprise. I learned that on the other side of resistance, there is discovery.

What did I discover in this case? Well, when I finally gave up trying to do mentally taxing tasks, I stumbled upon one thing that my brain could actually handle—music! From that point onwards, music became an incredible source of release for me. Some nights, when I faced terrifying episodes of shortness of breath, I would put on Italian music and allow myself to be moved by the bold tenor tones. Music helped calm me on difficult nights when I was all alone and struggling. It also helped me find some joy and inspiration in a time when so many other things had been taken away from me.

Too often we try to resist things, and that's what causes us angst. You might be sitting in traffic and be furious about it, even though getting worked up about the traffic is not going to help the cars around you move faster. Or you might get frustrated at your partner, your child, or a parent for a recurring flaw they exhibit even though your frustration is unlikely to change their behavior.

You can't always change your circumstances, but if you can develop a capacity to "be with what's so" exactly as it is, and exactly as it isn't, then you can find incredible freedom and power no matter what circumstances you face.[3]

And in that wide-open space, you might create room for something new to emerge.

Expect uncertainty

We live in an uncertain, ever-changing world, and yet we waste so much energy trying to chase certainty when it ultimately is never truly attainable!

In the early months of my illness, I jumped from doctor to doctor looking for a cure that would fix all my ailments. The challenge was that I was up to an impossible task. I was asking these doctors to give me a firm answer, when the reality at the time was that so much was still unknown about the virus.

The search for an answer started with optimism and ended with despair. Every time I would see a new doctor, I would have a skip in my step the day of the appointment thinking that: Today, I will finally get some answers. Then one of two things would occur. Either I would have the doctor tell me the truth, and offer me something to try but with the caveat that it may not work as a lot was still unknown; or I would have a doctor more confidently offer me a remedy, only to a discover a few days later that it wasn't the magic cure. Either way, the entire process was demoralizing.

After repeated cycles of ups and downs, I finally realized that my craving for a quick fix was not going to be satisfied. It was then that I began to open my eyes to the reality of the situation. From that point forward, instead of chasing certainty, I began to expect uncertainty.

This didn't mean giving up all hope, as I'm still an optimist at heart! It's just that I had to learn to balance my optimism with a good dose of hard truth. The reality I came to accept was that, while there were things I could try, there was no 100% guaranteed fix.

When I finally embraced this reality, I was able to accept uncertainty more powerfully. If a certain treatment didn't work, I wouldn't get as crushed as I did in the early days, because this time around, I went in with the expectation that it might work or it might not. The other thing that opened up once I embraced uncertainty was that instead of being attached to certain result, I was now much more committed to learning. If a certain treatment didn't work, instead of feeling completely dejected, I would get curious about why it didn't work, and figure out a new path forward.

So often, we are afraid of the unpredictable and are looking for someone, oftentimes an authority figure such as a doctor, politician, or senior leader in our organization, to give us all the answers. Then, when things don't go our way, we get to blame them. While this might give us a temporary scapegoat, it doesn't really help us in the long run.

Building our capacity to be with uncertainty takes some practice, but once we allow ourselves to get comfortable with discomfort, it's a much more empowering way to live.

3

Celebrate micro wins

Start small

There are endless ways to keep our bodies fit and strong, but what really helped me through this entire experience was focusing on a strong mind. After the days started blending into each other, I decided I needed practices to motivate myself. From that point on, I started setting micro-goals. On most days, these goals were simple and small. One morning, I would commit to eating a few bites of oatmeal so that I could take my medicine. The next day, I might step up to half a bowl. On more ambitious days, I would commit to writing a few words about my experience so that maybe I could help someone else who was suffering just like me. While these were small steps, they felt like victories and gave me something to look forward to.

Adopting these practices reacquainted me with the power of small steps in reaching big goals. Whether it's tackling a disease, committing to an exercise routine, building a writing habit, or any other pursuit, half the battle is just getting started. I have learned that taking on something for five minutes a day is better than setting goals so lofty that you never get started in the first place.

Celebrate small wins

On some days as I battled this disease, it felt like I was taking one step forward and two steps back, and it was easy to get overwhelmed by those setbacks. However, I soon realized that obsessing about disappointments was extremely demotivating. At the beginning of my illness, I was so overwhelmed by all the things that were not working that it was hard to notice when something was working. But as I progressed, I realized that celebrating wins was going to be absolutely necessary for my recovery.

I chose to focus more attention on the wins, even if they were very small to start, by adopting a practice that I learned with a team at work. Periodically, we sit down together and people celebrate themselves for something that they feel proud of from that day. It's a practice that takes some getting used to because most of us have not been trained to appreciate ourselves. However, in the later weeks of my battle, I decided to try it on and acknowledge myself for something at the end of each day. Usually, it was for a very small win—for example, that I mustered the energy to wash my bed sheets, or that I jumped back quickly from a setback earlier in the day. One day, my small win was that I made it outside for a walk to the pharmacy to get Pepto Bismol. Sometimes you just have to find humor, even in the dark moments!

An acknowledgment practice is not just a nice thing to do. It can have a profound impact on happiness and productivity. Neuroscience shows us that positive thoughts release serotonin, allowing us to feel happy, calmer, more emotionally stable, and less anxious. For me, this practice helped me temper my anxiety as I headed into the haunted nights.

What's more incredible is that building this practice over time can have real and lasting impacts. Research shows that such thinking can actually change neural pathways in the brain.

I've learned that picking a specific time in the day to celebrate these small wins can help build a rhythm. I do it right before bed, but you could also do it in your morning shower, while brushing your teeth, or on your daily commute. It may feel a little awkward at first because it's not something most of us are used to, but it's worth trying it on. After all, in these challenging times, we could all use a little more celebration in our lives!

Build lasting habits

Once you've had a few small wins, you can choose to turn these actions into ongoing habits. Habits require a lot of focus at first, but after a certain point, the behaviour that was so daunting at the start becomes automatic and effortless. Neuroscience shows us that one of the benefits of building habits is that, once you have repeated something many times, it gets infused into the circuitry of your brain; your brain then uses less energy to execute these habitual actions, freeing your mind up for other tasks.

Some people find it easy to develop habits. I personally am not a creature of habit, and so I have had to learn some "hacks" to help make habits stick in my life.

One of the habits I needed to develop when I returned back to work was learning how to take frequent mini-breaks. One of my doctors explained to me that, since my body had still not fully recovered yet, I would likely relapse without pacing and frequent rest. I soon learned that the doctor was very right. If didn't get enough rest, I would suffer from deep waves of fatigue and pain. I knew I had to follow the doctor's advice and take on a pacing strategy with breaks at frequent intervals, but the challenge was that this was very counter-intuitive to how I was used to working. Normally, I go full-out throughout the day. Now I had to learn to pause throughout the day to avoid severe flare-ups.

Building this new habit was challenging, and so I used some tricks I had accumulated over the years. The first thing I did was write down my intention clearly on a whiteboard right in front of my work area. Research shows that we're 20-40% more likely to achieve our goals if we picture them vividly or write them down. In big, bold letters, I wrote: "Pause before

the pain starts." Then I visualized myself pausing ev-
eryday and going outside for a mid-day walk in the
park.

In the growing body of research around habit
formation, one highly touted strategy is to build a
"habit streak," so I would try to go for as many days as
I could without breaking my mid-day walking habit.
For the early weeks, I needed to keep the reminder
up on my whiteboard; after a while, the value of these
breaks became so clear to me, that my walking shoes
began to go on without much thought!

Another trick I used to solidify this habit was tell-
ing a close work colleague about it. The act of declar-
ing a commitment out loud to another person makes
it more real. It also helped that my colleague would
ask me from time to time if I was taking enough
breaks, and gently call me out if she saw me pushing
myself too hard. I have found that having an account-
ability partner or a supportive community can be ex-
tremely powerful in building new habits.

Finally, I learned that we have to be generous
with ourselves when developing new practices. Just
like a child who is learning to ride a bicycle, it is al-
most certain that you will stumble or wipe out a few
times as you learn something new! Often, when we

fail at something, we tell ourselves, *I failed*, and that makes it much harder to recover. The alternative is to just get curious and playfully say to ourselves: *Well, that didn't seem to work today. I wonder why not? What might I try differently tomorrow?* And then, just like a child learning to ride a bike, we too can get back up again and not let one mishap kill our confidence.

No matter how big our aspirations are, we can make progress toward our goals if we give ourselves permission to take small steps and be gentle with ourselves along the way.

4

Embrace suffering

Accept suffering

All of us will endure suffering at some point in our lives. We will face heartbreak or betrayal, confront health issues, and lose loved ones. This is all part of the natural cycle of life, and yet we spend much of our lives trying to resist suffering rather than accepting it. The reality is that our time on earth is filled with many seasons, some brimming with joy and others laden with hardship.

Just a few months before I fell ill with this virus, I had the opportunity to attend a seven-day silent meditation retreat in Thailand. I was very intimidated by the idea of seven days of silence because up until that point in my life, all I had managed was ten minutes of meditation a day, and even that was challenging for me! Looking back though, taking on this challenge was a really good decision. While I could never have predicted it then, the lessons I learned at this silent retreat ended up being vitally helpful as I battled this crazy virus.

During the retreat, we would spend hours each day in meditation, sitting in silence on the wooden floor of a serene meditation hall atop a forested hill. During one session, I became painfully aware of a chronic pain pulsing in the left side of my lower back. When you're sitting still for hours a day, it's hard not to notice every little thing, and this pain started bothering me more than ever before. However, the instruction from the Buddhist monk was that no matter what pain you were feeling, try not to move positions to make the pain go away. His teaching was that pain is transient; that just as it comes, it will also eventually go.

For the first few days, I just couldn't follow those instructions. When I felt pain come, I would shift positions if it got very intense. Finally, after a few days, I surrendered to the monk's teachings and just let the pain be there while I sat still. After a while, I found that it did indeed disappear, or at least, my attention on it dissipated. What I discovered through this small action was a microcosm of a much larger teaching— that just like pain, everything in life will come and go, and that we can find some relief from suffering when we give up clinging to a fixed notion of how life should be.

Let go of unnecessary suffering

Over the past few months, I have definitely endured my share of pain. Some of this pain has been physical in nature, like pounding headaches, nauseating stomach pains, and a chronic feeling of constriction in my chest.

But I also discovered that much of my suffering was unnecessary, like the mental anguish I faced when trying to focus through brain fog or the suffering I endured lying awake at night wondering how my family would react if the worst should happen to me. I call this suffering unnecessary because all my worrying couldn't change these situations. Contemplating them might give me new insight, but worrying endlessly about them wouldn't change a thing.

It made me wonder: just how much of our lives do we spend suffering unnecessarily? How much time do we spend beating ourselves up? Sitting in guilt or shame? Feeling angry with others for things they may not have even intended? Worrying about circumstances that cannot be changed?

One question you might ask yourself when you're suffering is: "Will worrying about this actually change things?" If the answer is "no," then try and steer yourself back to the present, focus on what you actually can control, and learn to accept the things that you cannot change. I'm beginning to see that our time on earth is finite, and can imagine far better ways to use this precious time than worrying about things beyond our control!

Find strength in suffering

Many years ago, in my college dorm room, I had a Nietzsche quote on my wall: *"That which does not kill us makes us stronger."* Looking back at my life, I realize that my greatest bursts of personal growth have often come from my most difficult moments. What if, instead of seeing suffering as something terrible, we saw it as access to something more beautiful, as a gateway to growing our resilience and fortitude?

While I was battling this virus, a colleague of mine introduced me to an app that sent motivational quotes to my phone every few hours. The app had an uncanny ability to send me the exact quote I needed at that very moment. I remember one particular day that I was starting to feel sorry for myself and was about to enter into a vicious cycle of unnecessary suffering. Suddenly, I heard a *ping* on my phone and looked to see the quote: "Instead of 'why me?', say 'try me!'" I stopped and laughed out loud and then embraced that as my motto for the rest of the day. "Bring it on! Just try me!"

To build our own resilience to suffering, it's helpful to learn from the stories of those before us who have triumphed even when the odds were stacked against them. Early in my battle with this virus, during semi-lucid moments, I listened to the audiobook *Man's Search for Meaning* by Viktor Frankl[4]. This autobiographical tale recalls the life of Frankl, a Holocaust survivor who moved around to four different labor camps, including Auschwitz, and survived by finding meaning in his suffering.

One day, after a severe bout of intense gastrointestinal symptoms had completely eviscerated my appetite and left me unable to keep down food, I felt weak to my core. For a fleeting moment, I just wanted to give up. But then I thought of Frankl and so many others around the world battling hardship under more dire circumstances. I stopped feeling sorry for myself and recalled Frankl's wise words: *"Everything can be taken from a man but one thing: the last of the human freedoms—to choose one's attitude in any given set of circumstances, to choose one's own way."* I love these words, though for myself, I added "woman" to that sentence!

Suffering helps us learn what we are capable of because it pushes us to new limits. One of the symptoms I faced in the initial months was a disruption to my sleep cycle. For many days in a row, I would only get 2-3 hours of sleep, and some nights I might not get any sleep at all. This really pushed me to my limits because sleep is so critical to health on a normal day, and it's even more important when your body needs to heal.

In the early days of having sleep issues, I did not deal with it well. I had trouble functioning, was groggy and moody throughout the day, and felt like I had no control over things. Over time, however, I learned how to operate with less sleep. I also became more aware of my mood, and gained a better sense of when I could power through versus when I needed to stop and rest during the day. I was also very lucky to have a supportive co-worker whom I trust dearly who would gently call me out if she saw me operating from a state that wasn't my best; that would be a cue for me to take a step back until I was able to get some rest again.

What's fascinating is that even after my sleep returned, the heightened self-awareness I developed during the sleepless nights stayed with me. I am now a lot more aware of my emotional state, and have learned some strategies to pause and step away if I find myself operating from a stressed state.

Unlock empathy

Another beautiful thing about suffering is that it allows us to connect with others. When we begin to realize that we are not unique in our suffering, we might see that suffering need not be a solo act. In embracing those who are suffering alongside us, we may even find suffering to be a gateway to empathy. When I was struggling with brain fog, I felt connected in an entirely new way to all the elderly who are facing dementia. And when I could barely move a step, I found myself more aware of the plight of those who have mobility issues. I can't begin to claim to ever truly understand the experience of someone else, but I do think that suffering can strip away the noise that disconnects us, and in turn, activate our humility and empathy.

One choice we get to make is whether to open up or close down in times of suffering. If we close down, we risk feeling resentful, angry and alone, and we may end up lashing out in destructive ways at others, and even ourselves, to deal with our pain and isolation. However, if we allow ourselves to use our pain to open up and connect with others around us, we might discover that we are never truly alone.

Every moment provides an opportunity to turn toward others or turn away from them. In times of struggle, it's so easy sometimes to want to hunker down and hide. I remember days when I was struggling so much that I wanted to completely shut myself off from the world. Luckily, I had a friend who reached out to me daily to check in. Every time she reached out, I had a choice: *Do I turn toward her? Or do I turn away?* My friend's caring and reliable presence led me to turn toward her every time, and I am so glad I did because I always felt much better when I chose connection over isolation.

Going forward, when I next come across someone who is struggling, I just hope I can be the same kind of friend to them, one that invites them to turn toward, rather than turn away, in the time they need human connection the most.

5

Break free of limiting stories

Notice your inner monologue

Our minds are constantly filled with thoughts. We are either thinking about something that happened earlier in the day, or something about to happen. Or we're thinking about someone who upset us, or some judgment about ourselves. Most of us are not even aware of all the energy we spend on this internal chatter, and how it subconsciously runs our lives.

If you take a moment right now and listen to your thoughts, you will start hearing that internal monologue. For me, that internal monologue over the past months often sounded like, "I feel miserable right now," or "You just don't understand what I'm going through," or "Will I ever break free of this?"

It's not abnormal at all to have this barrage of thoughts. In fact, we can't control all the thoughts that pop into our minds. However, we can control how we relate to them. Meditation is one great practice for calming the mind and allowing us to observe our thoughts and feelings from a distance. If you're intimidated by meditation, simple practices like taking just a few deep breaths every now and then can also help declutter an anxious mind.

Science shows us why this is so powerful. When your mind perceives a threat, it triggers the body's sympathetic nervous system, elevating your heart rate, blood pressure, and fight-or-flight responses. Conversely, deep breathing activates your parasympathetic nervous system, enabling calm and clarity. Deep breathing helps signal to your body that you are no longer under threat.

Many nights, I would be jolted awake with a racing heart rate. In these moments, before I was even fully conscious, my automatic thought would be, *Why is this happening again?* Over time, I learned that the best way to handle these unpleasant awakenings was to take a few deep breaths until I felt calm again. Breathing helped me slow down my heart rate and get centered. It also helped me break free of the unhelpful thoughts swirling around in my head and come back to the present moment.

These practices of breathing and meditation didn't only help me in my battle with this virus, they also proved useful in other settings. When I returned to work, if I had a difficult encounter with someone, I would try to pause and take a few deep breaths before going on to the next task or meeting. So often we have a disruptive event happen to us early in the day, like a squabble with a partner, a frustrating meeting, or getting caught in bad morning traffic, and then we carry that with us throughout the day.

I think the reason we're so often exhausted by the end of the day is that we drag unresolved issues from morning to night along with us like a heavy bag of bricks! I am fully guilty of this myself, especially times when I've packed my days without any space to pause. Luckily though, by building small practices into our daily routines, like taking three deep breaths before a meeting or task, we can find a little more peace in our days.

Let go of limiting stories

Once I had gotten through the initial few weeks of battling this virus, I thought I was over the worst part. However, in the months that followed, I was faced with an even more daunting prospect. I read that if symptoms don't improve in six months, there is a high likelihood that the post-viral symptoms can turn into a more permanent chronic illness. This was completely terrifying to me.

Luckily, in the weeks that followed the most acute phase of this illness, I started to improve week by week. While progress was slow, I still felt hopeful since things were moving in the right direction. However, a few months in, everything changed. One day, as I was walking to the pharmacy to pick up medicine, I found myself desperately short of breath again even though the pharmacy is just a five-minute walk from my house.

In the weeks that followed, many of the symptoms that I thought I had beaten for good came back again in full force. The waves of fatigue became so intense again that I would have to lie down to rest in the middle of work just to make it through the day. Up until that point, I had been convinced that I could beat this thing eventually, but in those subsequent weeks when my health worsened, I started to lose hope.

The thought that this condition might never go away was extremely depressing. The physical torture was bad enough, but the mental anguish made things even worse. I soon realized that I couldn't keep going on like this. That's when I was reminded of a practice I had been trained in through my work in conscious leadership. The practice is to separate "what actually happened" from "what we make it mean." The idea here is that sometimes our brains automatically ascribe meaning to a situation, but that meaning might not be the truth.[5]

I sat down and noticed what was actually happening. I tried to focus only on facts that could be objectively observed. For example, I noticed that when I walked up a hill, I would get short of breath and have pains in my upper left chest. Or that the night before, I woke up at 2 a.m. with a heart rate of 150 beats per minute.

And then I noticed what I made all of this mean. Every time those symptoms flared, my brain automatically made it mean that, given that I was now past the six-month point, I was likely facing a permanent condition.

However, when I separated "what happened" from "what I made it mean," I realized that a lot of my assumptions might not be true at all. For example, the assertion that those who have symptoms for more than six months are likely to face chronic illness was just a claim about what might be true in the average case and didn't necessarily apply to me. And the story going off in my head that I would never recover from my latest relapse wasn't necessarily true either. After all, I had recovered from relapses before!

So often, we get trapped in automatic thought patterns that lead us to believe that there is only one way out. When we constrain ourselves to a fixed interpretation of a situation, it closes us down from seeing the multiple possibilities that might exist.

Once I had this epiphany, I felt like I had my power back in the situation. The first thing I did was call my doctor and explain the situation, and she offered me a new course of treatment to try. The second thing I did was to become more conscious of how I responded to the pain when it came back. When it did, if my mind began to fixate on worries about becoming chronically ill, I would force myself to interrupt those thoughts and instead say, "All that is happening right now is that my heart is beating at 150 beats per minute. I will be okay. I have techniques that I have learned to slow down my heart rate." And then I would focus on getting better in that moment vs. letting my mind spiral. What I found was that, as I started to get more skilled at interrupting automatic thought patterns, I felt much more powerful in dealing with difficult situations. The pain didn't disappear, but I was able to handle it better.

This tool of separating "what happened" from "what we make it mean" can be used in so many situations in our lives. How many of us have heard an offhand comment from a spouse or family member or work colleague, and then made up a whole story about what it means about us or about them? We are constantly living in our stories. However, when we jump from assumptions to conclusions without inquiring about what else might be happening in that situation, we limit ourselves. When we get curious instead, we can break free of these limiting stories, and rediscover our power again.

Use your words wisely

Another technique to escape limiting stories is to notice our language. The words we use with others matter, and so do the words we say to ourselves! In the early days of this virus, if I woke up feeling ill in the morning, I might tell myself: "Oh no, this is going to be a bad day!" The problem with words like "bad day" is that by saying them, they now become the frame through which we see everything. Pretty soon, we start paying extra attention to all the bad things that happen, and in doing that, we make ourselves powerless for the entire day.

However, we do have a choice in the language we use. Once I realized that, I began to tweak my words slightly. Instead of saying, "This is a bad day," I'd say, "Right now, I am having an 'off' moment." That small shift in language let me be honest about what was happening in that moment without throwing the whole day into the trash. This little trick worked so beautifully that I put up a note for myself with the words "It's okay to have an 'off' moment" near my workspace so that I could see it every day. That helped me catch myself anytime I started falling into the "bad day" trap!

So often, we use language unintentionally, and in doing so, create conditions that leave us resigned and cynical. What might be possible if we were all a bit more intentional about our language? If we truly understood how our words can actually shape everything around us?

When we get the potential of language as a generative force, not only can we use it to help us in times of trouble, we can also use it as a tool to create new things in the world. When John F. Kennedy declared to the world that we would land a man on the moon by the end of the decade, it awakened the imagination of many, and his words created a new reality. Malala Yousafzai, the young Pakistani advocate for girls' education, is another leader who evokes a sense of possibility through her words, inspiring hope in a new generation of activists. Malala recently spoke at a virtual global convening hosted by my workplace and I was so moved by what she shared: *"What I have learned through my activism is that the voice of one girl can be really powerful; that it can scare people with guns."*

Oftentimes, when we think about creative people, we imagine artists or musicians and might say to ourselves, "I don't have those talents, so I'll never be creative." Yet if we truly understood the generative nature of our words, we would discover that every single one of us has the power to create.

PART II

REDISCOVER JOY

6

Slow down and soak it in

Notice what's right there

Like many New Yorkers, I lead a busy life. Being sick forced me to slow down and take life in. In the first months of my illness, every night at 7 p.m., I would pull myself out of bed, open my window, take in a breath of fresh air, and clap for the frontline workers. I have taken thousands of breaths in my life, but until then, I had never really fully soaked them in like this.

Sometimes, as I slowed down, emotions of fear, sadness and anger rose to the surface. However, as

I allowed all my emotions to bubble up, I also had a pleasant surprise. Instead of being solely overwhelmed with difficult emotions, I found my heart opening up to all the love, connection, and beauty that surrounded me.

As one example, seven weeks into my fight, I celebrated my 40th birthday. On paper, that day might have sounded like a disaster. There was no big celebration. And yet, it was the most beautiful birthday ever. As I received warm notes from friends and family around the world, something amazing happened. Instead of the day whizzing by, I was able to really sit with all the love that was pouring in. I didn't let it pass me by. I soaked it all in. It was a deeply moving experience.

Slowing down also helped me rediscover things I had taken for granted. When I left my apartment after 27 days in isolation, the first thing I noticed were the beautiful tulips growing in a little patch outside of my building. I have lived in this apartment for five years. Why had I never really noticed these flowers in springtime before? Oh, and the feeling of a breath of fresh air, a gust of wind, and the first time seeing trees again after a month indoors! It was as if I were a kid experiencing these things for the first time. What would life feel like if we always approached the world with childlike wonder? What if we soaked in the magic of each moment like it was our first and last one on earth? Instead of taking these simple pleasures for granted, what if we were truly present in our lives?

Learning to savor the good experiences in life is one of the most important keys to well-being. Several studies suggest that gratitude can have a positive impact on physical health and psychological well-being. Those who are more grateful are also found to be happier, more satisfied with their lives, less materialistic, and less likely to suffer from burnout.

But busyness has become a normal way of life. In fact, we often wear it as a badge of honor. We are so busy running on autopilot, often in triggered states, that we can easily miss what's right in front of us. We miss the magic that exists simply in taking a walk or opening our hearts to the love in our life. We rush through that morning embrace with a partner or child as routine, rather than squeezing every ounce of joy from those precious moments.

Slowing down helped me pause and notice. I am now so much more aware of what's been right in front of me all along.

Unlearn bad habits

Slowing down didn't just help me savor the little things in life. It also forced me to recognize the importance of rest. In battling post-viral fatigue syndrome, I learned that if I didn't pause and rest regularly, I would quickly relapse.

So when I returned to work, I had to learn entirely new ways of operating. I had to say no to meetings and projects that I would have otherwise taken on. I had to pause in the middle of the day and take a rest in order to keep waves of pain and fatigue from escalating. I had to learn that while I was brimming with ambition around things I wanted to accomplish, not everything had to get done that day. And most of all, I had to learn to let go of any guilt associated with operating slowly, because the guilt just made the mental and physical pain worse. On my fridge, I put a Post-it Note with the words "Be gentle with yourself" as a daily reminder to practice self-compassion. Soon I discovered that when I was kind and respectful to myself, I was also much more grounded and generous in my interactions with others around me.

Slowing down is hard for so many of us "achievers" because our default norms are set otherwise. Initially, I tried to "power through" the fatigue and pain.

But for the first time in my life, that strategy did not work. What I discovered about slowing down is that it's not really about learning a new skill; rather, it's about unlearning.

When our routines are turned upside down, it can be daunting, that's for sure. Yet disruptive moments like this one are also a perfect time to break free of default ways of being. We can start questioning the things we do on autopilot and focus instead on the things that really matter.

Be present

In the early days of this illness, when deep bouts of fatigue kept me bedridden, I remember how much joy I took in finally being able to stand up and just make my bed (even if sometimes I would get back into it 10 minutes later!). In my normal life, making my bed is a task I do automatically without even thinking about it. But over the past few weeks, I have taken on this activity, and so many other activities like walking and eating, with greater intentionality, focusing on being fully present rather than letting these moments just pass me by.

This unprecedented era is inviting us all to be more mindful in our daily actions. Previously, we may have traveled from place to place without thinking much about it. Now, the simple act of leaving the house, putting on a mask, and ensuring we don't put others and ourselves at risk is something we have to be intentional about. In a similar light, we have the opportunity in this moment to be more mindful about so many other aspects of our lives, including how we interact with the people around us.

I am deeply aware that isolation can be deadly for so many who are less fortunate, so I don't claim that these new opportunities are possible for everyone, especially those who are struggling to just survive. But for those who have their basic needs met, I think we have a responsibility to open our eyes to the gift that this era is giving us. What a shame it would be to come to the end of our lives and discover that we missed appreciating the "little things" that feel so ordinary at times—like a daily embrace with our partner—to later realize that these were the "big things" after all.

.

7

Awaken untapped senses

Activate your soul

We all need things that energize our souls. In the early days of this virus, when my brain was too foggy to do anything else, music was my savior. It helped me leave my small New York apartment and escape to another world! Some nights, I would put on an uplifting song and imagine myself running up a mountain in Nepal I had visited a couple years back. I would visualize myself standing at the summit breathing in the fresh air with a 360 view of the stunning Himalayas. In this, I found some peace.

Another thing that was critical to my recovery was laughter. A wise friend of mine who had gone through a very difficult tragedy of his own shared with me once that humor got him through the darkest of times, so I tried to find some light and laughter every day, even if just for a few moments. Some days, I got a good laugh watching funny videos of my nieces and nephews that my brother or sister would send me. On other days, I used ridiculous Bitmojis to convey my moods so that I would get a little chuckle even when I was feeling miserable.

A good friend also got me into watching funny old movies like *Roman Holiday* that made me laugh out loud. Sitting alone in silence all day, I got more sensitive to sound, and so it was especially nice to hear the sound of my own roaring laughter from time to time. Often in our daily lives, we get so caught up in our day-to-day routines that life gets overly serious. I think we can all learn something from children and remember to be playful with life and laugh out loud as much as we can!

For me, music and laughter activated my soul. For others, this joy comes from baking, dancing, nature, writing, poetry, running, family time, social gatherings, or quiet time. Oftentimes, what stirs our souls are the activities we enjoyed as children but put aside as we got busy living our "adult" lives.

We can find so much joy in our lives if we allow ourselves to indulge in play. Yet it's easy to neglect this part of our lives with excuses such as, "I don't have time," or "This feels indulgent," or "I need to be productive all the time." The truth is that we can always make a little time for play even if it means starting small. We just have to give ourselves permission for it, because we've conditioned ourselves to think that play is only for children. Yet studies have shown that play can be powerful for adults too in so many ways, including enhancing our problem solving abilities, creativity, and connection.

After I discovered my love for music again, I borrowed a friend's guitar and started learning how to play. At first, I would only spend five minutes a day playing because I too initially got caught up in thinking, *This is not productive, and I have so much else to do.* Very soon, however, I started making more time to play because it brought me so much joy. When we connect with the things that bring us light, I find that we can be quite resourceful in making them happen, even in the face of constraints.

Whatever it is that nourishes you, find it and re-connect to it! If we don't indulge our souls every once in a while, then what's the point of living anyway?

Nourish your body

By the third week of this illness, I had lost 10 lb or nearly 10% of my body weight. I had zero appe-tite but knew that I needed energy, and so I had to force myself to eat. The challenge was that no matter how much I needed nourishment, my body simply wouldn't accept food.

What's fascinating is that when I finally started craving food again in the fourth week, all I wanted were greens and fruits. It's like my body was sending me a message: "You've been ignoring me, now give me some real nourishment, please!" How ironic that when I finally needed to put on weight, instead of craving ice cream, all I wanted was salad!

In the subsequent days, I had one focus: Gain weight! Like many women, gaining weight has never been my goal, so I found it amusing that I was count-ing calories to make sure I was eating enough, not the other way around. When my body was withering

away, though, all I could think to myself is how ridic-
ulous this fixation with body issues is in our society.
Yes, I absolutely want a strong, healthy, fit body and
have always been committed to healthy eating and
regular exercise in pursuit of that. However, what's
silly to me now is how much attention we devote
to having the "perfect" body. Ninety-nine percent
of people will never attain the image that we see in
magazines (nor should they!), and the mental energy
this obsession consumes could be used for far better
purposes. Imagine what could be accomplished with
the millions of collective hours of energy we could
repurpose if we weren't obsessing about our weight
and looks.

All this being said, I could not ignore my diet while
I was sick. In fact, focusing on nutritional intake was
extremely important for my healing. What's surpris-
ing, though, is that being sick completely changed my
relationship with food. Eating was no longer about
satisfying a sweet craving, avoiding the boredom of a
mid-day slump, or an excuse to socialize with friends
on a Saturday night. Instead, my food intake became
purely about healing my body, for example, ensuring
that I was getting enough protein to rebuild my mus-
cles, or enough magnesium to strengthen my heart.

Don't get me wrong: I'm a "foodie" who enjoys all the rich cuisines that New York has to offer. However, these weeks of approaching food as nourishment rather than as a pleasure source made me much more mindful of what I was putting in my body. Before this illness, I'd always known in my head that I "should" eat healthy and tried to do so for the most part, but admittedly I did cheat from time to time!

This experience changed something in me, though. Since my body was so fragile, I could actually feel myself getting weaker on days when I wasn't as conscious about what I was putting into it. Now, I'm no longer driven by a feeling that I "should be" healthy. Rather, through this very visceral experience, I have a deeper intuitive sense now of how my choice of food on any given day can completely alter my physical and mental energy.

The other thing I discovered is how important movement is both for the body and soul. On nights when I was too anxious to sleep, I would get up and pace around my apartment—a form of walking meditation I learned in Thailand—and it would help calm my restless mind. Most people associate meditation with sitting cross-legged and doing deep breathing, but I have found that walking, swimming, running

and other forms of movement can be equally power-
ful ways to clear the mind. After 27 days, when I was fi-
nally allowed to go outside for real walks, the feeling of
being fully in motion again brought me so much joy.

We can also add a little fun to movement! There
were many days when I faced fatigue and body aches
so severe that all I wanted to do was lie in bed. I knew,
though, that I had to get moving to avoid the risk of
pneumonia and other infections. So I adopted a little
practice I learned from my nieces in London and put
on a Bollywood bhangra tune (aptly named "Radha
on the Dance Floor") at full volume on loudspeak-
ers first thing in the morning. When just a moment
before, the fatigue had been so intense that I didn't
think it was possible to even lift a toe out from under-
neath my bed covers, a few minutes after the music
went on, I found myself magically rising (or some-
times bopping!) out of bed.

Embrace the mind-body connection

In battling this illness, I also learned how to better
listen to my body. After a few weeks of checking my
vitals daily, I developed the uncanny ability to guess
my temperature or heart rate even before the moni-
tor showed a result. On the sage advice of my mother,

I also learned not to fight the fatigue but rather take it as a sign that my body needed more rest.

I have always believed that the mind-body connection is important, but I clearly remember the day this really came alive for me. I was sitting at home and got a call from the doctor's office that the blood work I had done earlier that week was invalid because it had been mishandled en route to the lab. I was livid! I hate having blood drawn, and it had taken every ounce of energy in me to give that blood because I was already so weak. I was furious that it had been lost.

What happened the next moment was intense. Less than a few seconds after receiving that phone call, my heart rate shot up 50 beats per minute. I know because I was wearing a heart-rate monitor and also because I could viscerally feel my already unstable heart pumping even harder. In that moment, I really got how much our thoughts affect our bodies. It took me a few moments to settle down again, but from that point forward, I was much more aware of how my anger and stress could negatively impact my health.

Our bodies hold incredible wisdom, but we've lost our capacity to listen to them, and I believe we could gain a lot if we rediscover this ability. There is a whole field of work called "somatics" that trains people to get in tune with their bodies so they can notice how stress lives in their bodies and learn how to use movement to release it. Studies have shown that somatic work can help those who have suffered from traumatic experiences, including veterans and victims of abuse.

Even if we have not suffered from major trauma, all of us could benefit from getting more in tune with our bodies, even in small ways. Imagine, for example, if you were better at noticing early warning signs of stress when walking into a difficult interaction with a colleague or loved one. Being more aware of a clenched jaw or tight shoulders might be just the signal you need to pause, center yourself, and re-engage once you're in a less triggered state.

Under stress, we all regress. We go into automatic responses, often ones we have been conditioned to embody from a young age when we first encountered stress. This affects us physically as our heart rates and stress hormones shoot up. When we were young, these responses might have been justified in response to the threats we were facing. The challenge is that, we've often hung on to these automatic reactions many years later. Our bodies continue to go into fight-or-flight mode when we perceive a threat, even though it's no longer a real threat. So the work for us now becomes learning how to interrupt these habituated patterns.

If you don't pause in those moments of stress, you may find yourself interacting with others from an agitated state and come to regret your words and actions later. The more adept you get at noticing these early signals in your body, the better you can become at engaging with others from a spacious state rather than from your most regressive state.

A doctor friend of mine shared with me a tool that she learned as part of a mindfulness training called "Two Feet, One Breath." Before entering a patient's room, the doctor is invited to take a moment to pause, feel both feet on the floor, inhale and exhale, come into the present moment, and then use that presence to connect with the patient. I love the simplicity of this practice, which makes it accessible to anyone. It could be something to try standing at your front door right before re-entering your home after a long day; or in the morning, right before waking up your kids; or as a pause moment between meetings or other events in the day. There are many other mindfulness practices that we can use to further grow our mind-body connection, from mindful eating to mindful walking, once we understand how powerful this connection truly is.

My final discovery throughout this illness was how much I missed human touch. It's funny the things we don't even value until they are taken away from us. Some nights I just craved someone by my bedside to hold my hand or give me a tight embrace. I kept thinking to myself, *When I am fully recovered, I want to go around to nursing homes where so many elderly are battling this horrid illness all alone and just give the residents big hugs.* Maybe "professional hugger" will become my new calling on weekends!

But seriously, no one should suffer this crazy illness alone without a little human touch. And we should all remember to be a bit more present with the embraces we do have.

8

Simplify and be free

Declutter your space

What a simple existence I lived the first month of battling this virus! My time in isolation reminded me of my week of silent meditation in Thailand. There, I lived an extremely minimalist life. I slept on a wooden slab with a bamboo mat in a shared room with 30 other people. There were no electronic devices, books, music, conversations, or any other form of stimulation allowed. We ate two meals a day of soup broth and fresh vegetables and fasted for 16 hours.

The rest of the time was mostly spent in hour-long intervals of sitting and walking meditation. I won't lie. The experience was agonizing at first, especially for someone who was used to always being on the go, mentally and physically.

However, as the days went on, I found peace in the simplicity of it all. Since all my possessions for that week could fit into a small backpack, I didn't have to make many decisions. I would wear one pair of clothes one day, and then scrub them down with soap and hang them to dry while I wore the second set the following day. Toward the end of the week, because my mind was less cluttered, I had fewer cravings. At the beginning of the week, I would load up on food at lunchtime to prepare for 16 hours of fasting; by the end of the week, I would feel satisfied with just a ladleful of soup. Because my mind was so free, I didn't have physical cravings anymore.

While my experience in quarantine with this virus was not exactly the same as this austere retreat, there were many parallels. I didn't need much stuff, just a couple sets of comfortable clothes, a simple diet, some basic hygiene products, a bed, and that's about it. Okay, well, my iPhone did still come in handy for music and staying connected! But beyond that, there was very little I needed.

Now I'm not saying we need to go to that extreme in everyday life. But there is something about our rampant consumerism that is deeply disconcerting. The idea that if we just have more stuff, we will be happy is so prevalent in our society and yet so dangerous. We collect possessions thinking they will make us happy, and perhaps they might for a little while, but that happiness is fleeting. Material goods are necessary up until a certain level. I recognize that many people in the world are not fortunate enough to live at this level, and that is a real concern. But for those whose basic needs have been met, I believe that what we're really yearning for is a deep inner peace that excess consumption will never fully satisfy.

Minimalist living also taught me to be less wasteful, which I think is a conversation we should all seriously engage in if we want to leave a habitable planet behind for the next generation. Living in a big city with a rampant consumerist culture, it's easy to indulge in behaviors that contribute to the destruction of our planet. Yet it's clear that's not sustainable, and that we all have a responsibility here.

One good thing that has come out of lockdowns is that we're actually witnessing how a pause in our excessive habits can make a difference to our environment. In many polluted cities around the world, air quality dramatically improved when activity was shut down. And there was a mass reduction in ground and air travel that's sparking questions about how we might embrace lower levels of travel even when this pandemic dies down. Of course, lockdowns are not the answer, as we have to ensure that people can earn livelihoods. However, my hope is that when restrictions ease, we don't just return to "business as usual" but instead use what we have learned to create more sustainable ways of living so we can leave a habitable planet for future generations.

Declutter your mind

My sister is the amazing mother of four kids under the age of 10. When the pandemic first hit London, where she lives, schools closed for a while, so she had all her kids at home. I asked her if the kids missed school, and she shared that they did miss their friends, but she also noticed that they seemed freer in this new era. They had more time to play without an agenda and to use their imaginations.

In the same way, I think this pandemic has created space for many of us to pause. I believe that it is in these spaces that the deepest reflection can happen—when we allow ourselves to not schedule every moment of every day, when we free ourselves from the need to be productive and efficient all the time, when we can go for a walk just for the sake of going for a walk, and when we can put down our smartphones and let our minds wander a little.

So many great novelists, scientists, artists and other great minds got bursts of creative inspiration when they allowed themselves to daydream and let their minds wander. I was glad to have this time to let my mind wander in ways that I hadn't allowed for before in my busy lifestyle.

One habit I have developed over the past few months is going for a daily walk. My doctor prohibited me from doing any exercise beyond this, but I have come to really appreciate these walks, not just for the physical activity but also for the mental clarity they provide. Some days, I listen to a podcast or audiobook, but many other days, I wander without any agenda and embrace the free-flowing energy that emerges.

One day, as I was on my daily walk in the park, a tree that looked like it must be at least a hundred years old captured my attention. As I stared at the roots, I began wondering about the tree's history. And that sparked a thought for me about my own history and all the ancestors who had come before me. So later that week, I started asking my mother questions about our family history, and what I learned was fascinating.

I grew up in Canada around a lot of extended family on my dad's side. Most of them pursued careers in business and entrepreneurship, and so I always felt a bit of the odd one out pursuing my calling in education. However, as I dug into my family's history, a revelation I had was that on my mom's side, I actually come from a long line of educators. It is something that I had never reflected on before but was excited to discover, given my own passion for and commitment to education.

I learned that my great-grandfather's brother had traveled as a cook on a ship from India to Uganda at the age of 12, and then later returned to India where he opened up a school for girls at a time when it was pretty progressive to invest in girls' education. I also learned of my maternal grandmother's time as a headmistress at a school in Kenya. And I got re-connected to my aunt who runs an amazing Saturday school in London that helps kids grow as compassionate leaders who can be of service to others. All these years, I had never taken enough time to fully ask the questions like: "Where do I come from? How am I connected to my ancestors? What have I inherited from those who have come before me?"

I wonder what else we would all discover if we gave ourselves more space to let go of our busy agendas and just let our minds wander a little like we used to do as children.

Some other questions I've been wondering about recently include: How could I spend more of my time on the things I love, and less time on things that drain my energy? How might I show up calmly all the time, even on days when everything around me seems chaotic? How do I live into my core value of "being generous" with every single person, even those who frustrate or anger me? What's the one thing I can do today that would make the biggest contribution to the impact I ultimately want to see in the world? And finally, how do I develop a deliberate practice to keep reflecting on these questions?

Less is more

Like many people, I struggle at times with prioritization, and tend to take on more than I can handle. Beyond feeling overwhelmed and exhausted, the greater consequence of this is that it robs us of devoting our energy to the things that we truly care about.

When I returned back to work, I was eager to come back in full force, but I soon learned that if I pushed myself too hard, I would relapse. So I had to take on less. Initially, the shift was difficult because I had to say no to things that I would have normally said yes to. At first, I had a lot of guilt around that. But with limited hours in the day, I had no choice but to prioritize the most important tasks, and learn to say no to everything else.

I have to say I'm grateful that this happened because it taught me a lot about how to manage my time and energy. When I first returned back to work, sometimes I would face such bad waves of fatigue and pain that I only had a few good working hours in the day. So I had to be ruthless about saying "no" to requests. What I realized from this was a really powerful lesson: when we're clear on what we want to say "yes" to (in this case, my health), it's a lot easier to say "no" to other things. Even as my health improves, I'm taking this valuable lesson with me.

The other thing I learned is that, when we're distracted, an hour can disappear into thin air; when we are fully present, an hour can go a long way. When I returned back to work, because I was deeply aware that my symptoms could flare up at any moment, one of my mottos became: "Don't waste the good moments." While I had fewer hours in the day when I felt physically well, I experienced those good moments much more fully. The irony is that, instead of time shrinking, it felt like time had actually grown because I was much more mindful with the time I did have.

I think our tendency to take on "more" comes from anxiety. We feel that we're not doing enough, or that we're not good enough, and so we take on more tasks to fill our days. If instead we can pause long enough to get clear on what's really essential, we can strip out a lot of clutter.

There are two simple practices I have learned to help me manage my energy and time. The first is pausing every once in a while to ask: "Why?" Children do this amazingly well! "Why are we doing this?" they might ask, or "Why does it matter?" If I ask myself "why" multiple times and am not clear on the answer, it's a clue that maybe what I'm doing in that moment is not so important to me.

A second practice is to be more aware of the stories we're telling ourselves. If I catch myself rushing around frantically saying, "I don't have enough time," I now try to interrupt those thoughts, and say instead, "I have enough. I am enough. All is well." It seems a bit silly at first to use these phrases, but if you allow yourself to give it a go, you might discover how powerful a simple switch in language is. It gets us out of fight-or-flight mode, and allows us to be okay with the time we do have.

In this fast-paced world, so many of us struggle with our relationship with time. We try to fix this with productivity hacks. However, I have found freedom with time actually comes through getting clear on what we want, letting go of guilt, and building our capacity to be present in the moment.

PART III

EMBRACE
INTERCONNECTEDNESS

9

Find your tribe

Find belonging in community

I love being exposed to people from different walks of life. At the same time, it's also nice sometimes to come home to a community where I feel completely at ease. In my regular life, I am fortunate to have more than one community where I feel deep belonging. Yet in the early weeks of battling this virus, I often felt alone, because it's hard for people to fully relate to something they haven't experienced themselves. I started wondering about who could relate and stumbled upon an online COVID-19 support group. In other words, I stumbled upon a new tribe for this harrowing time.

The first time I read online posts from this community, I almost cried with relief. For days, I had been questioning my own sanity and wondering if I was going crazy. But as I started reading these posts, I realized that there were so many others just like me dealing with strange symptoms that cycled through in waves. Posts such as:

"I'm at Day 43 and can't sleep for more than 3 hours at a time. Anyone else facing this? And what have you tried?"

"Have been sick for months and the main remaining symptoms now are crashing fatigue plus gastro symptoms, low-grade fevers, racing heart, and tingling body. I have tried working a few days, and then I needed to stay in bed for a week. Anyone else at this stage? What questions should I be asking the doctor?"

In reading those posts, for the first time, I didn't feel so alone anymore. In this one online community, there were thousands of other confused souls just like me who were wrestling with this strange virus and trying to make sense of it.

A tribe can be useful in many ways. It can be an incredible release when you feel a sense of belonging without having to explain or filter yourself. I remember one day in particular that I had an especially frustrating telehealth visit with a new doctor. From the beginning of the visit, I felt like the doctor was trying to chalk up my symptoms to anxiety. I felt minimized and frustrated throughout the visit and disheartened at being misdiagnosed.

Later that night, as I was browsing the online support group channels, I discovered that many others had experienced similar interactions with their doctors that left them feeling unheard. In that moment, I felt seen and understood, and that gave me the confidence to step out and try again. My next interaction with the doctor turned out to be more productive. However, I might not have found the strength for it had I not had a safe community to come to first where I could feel truly heard. There is nothing more powerful than being seen and heard, especially by those who share in your suffering.

Seek growth in community

The other benefit of a tribe is that it pushes your growth and learning. With the scarcity of information on COVID-19 in the early days of this virus, I found this online support group to be one of my greatest sources of information. For example, when I started suffering strange symptoms such as tingling and brain fog, I found a #neurological channel, where I was able to ask questions of others who were facing similar symptoms.

Or when the media kept saying that this disease only lasted 14 days, I found comfort in finding channels that were named #30+ days and #60+ days that helped me realize that there were other chronic sufferers just like me. Later, the media and medical community caught up and started reporting on the plight of the long-haulers, but that definitely was not the case in the early days of this virus.

In fact, the increased awareness about long COVID is the direct result of the leadership of a small group of people within this online community who were so frustrated by the lack of attention on long COVID that they decided to take matters into their own hands. They organized a detailed survey of members of this online community so they could inspire the medical research community to focus more attention on our plight. They then partnered with journalists to publish the first articles on long COVID, ultimately leading to greater media attention on long-haulers. I'm incredibly inspired by how this small group of determined people self-organized to raise attention for this neglected patient population that I now call my tribe.

My biggest takeaway from this experience is that whatever we're struggling with, we should remember that we're never really alone. There are likely hundreds, or sometimes millions of other human beings who are enduring or have endured similar suffering. While it's unbearable to imagine that so many others are struggling too, it's also quite comforting to not feel alone.

Whenever you find yourself in a difficult situation, remember that you might be able to find comfort and growth in community. It's so easy to feel alone sometimes, but that's exactly the time that it's most worth reaching out. A question to ask yourself when you're struggling is: "Who else in the world might be struggling with what I am dealing with, and can I find a community to support me?"

This can apply for personal struggles but also in our work lives. Early in my career, when I was operating in male-dominated environments, I noticed that sometimes in a business meeting, even if I was the most senior team member in the room, my clients might automatically turn to a more junior male team member. While this bias may have been unconscious, it was still something I needed to navigate. For too long, I struggled on my own to figure out how to handle these situations, not recognizing that there had been so many women before me who had faced similar scenarios. So now, when I feel stuck on a challenge, I always ask myself the question of who might have grappled with this before that I can learn from?

10

Make gratitude a habit

Notice the good stuff

In the past months, I have had so much gratitude for people in my life, close friends, family, and strangers alike. And with a lot of time to sit idle, I had space to really sit with this gratitude rather than letting it pass me by. I have enormous appreciation for my dear friend Sakshi, a frontline doctor, who made time to help me get medical treatment even when she herself was working 50 days in a row treating droves of patients at the peak of the pandemic. I am so grateful for my friend Wendy, whose steady warmth and wisdom brought me comfort on dark days and cheer to fight for brighter ones. And for my friend Aaron, who showed up in a heartbeat in the middle of the night to take me to the hospital. I am also grateful to my colleague Katherine, who supported me with such care when I came back to work, even when I was not my best self. And for my friend Sid, who kept me motivated to get this book done, even when the pain and fatigue felt all-consuming. I am also thankful for my family, who are always there for me without fail!

There were also many people who passed through my life just once but made such a difference. I remember Glenda, the woman who picked up the phone at the pharmacy and said assuredly, "Don't worry, honey, I got you!" when she heard how anxious I was that my delivery of blood thinners had gotten lost in transit. And Carl, the paramedic who took an extra moment to look me in the eyes and explain to me what was going on with my symptoms in a way that no one else had done before. And the kind ER nurse who had traveled to New York from Tulsa to provide extra coverage during the peak of the pandemic. And the list goes on and on and on. In fact, the list got so long that I started writing down names on my whiteboard in my kitchen so I didn't forget.

I think the act of simply noticing the good stuff is something we need to practice. We have become so inundated with bad news all around us, especially in the media, that I fear we have become overly cynical about life. This is understandable from an evolutionary perspective; in our hunter-gatherer days, our minds were wired to look out for threats as a mechanism for survival. However, in today's world, while we do not need to fight for survival in the same way, we have still retained these primal instincts of vigilance. This leads to a negativity bias that no longer serves us.

The good news is that we can rewire our brains simply by training ourselves to notice these positive events and hold them in our thoughts for a little while. Studies show that retraining our brains to focus on positive stimuli can make a real difference to our well-being. One leading researcher in the field of positive psychology, Dr. Martin E. P. Seligman, conducted a study where he asked participants to write and personally deliver a letter of gratitude to someone who has never been properly thanked for their kindness. Those who wrote these letters exhibited a huge increase in happiness scores, with benefits lasting for more than a month.[6]

Focusing on the good stuff has also been shown to have a profound impact on our brains and other physiological responses. In a 2017 study by Kyeong et al.[7], where participants were asked either to focus their attention on someone they love or on someone that makes them angry, the effects of these two interventions were captured by monitoring participants' heart rates and fMRI scans of the brain. The study showed that the first intervention lowered participants' heart rates in a way that correlated with stronger mental health. This intervention also had a positive effect on the amygdala, the brain's center for processing emotions and memories.

Given the tangible benefits of noticing the good stuff, it's well worth expanding our awareness to be more intentional. We can do this in many ways: by taking a moment each evening to silently reflect on what was good about that day; by keeping a gratitude journal where we write down a few good things from the day; or by cultivating other mindfulness practices that expand our ability to notice the beauty that's all around us.

Express appreciation

Noticing is the first step. Expressing it comes next. Why is it that we have trouble expressing our love and appreciation even when we feel immense gratitude for others? How silly is it that the most beautiful odes to people are delivered at their funerals when they can't appreciate them? Why not say these words directly to our loved ones when they are alive and well? Maybe we assume that people know how we feel. I know I have used that excuse many times. Of course, my friend/partner/family member/colleague knows how much I value them. How could they not? Isn't it obvious? But the truth is, while some of this can be felt, we could all probably get better at expressing our love for others.

The acknowledgment of another human being is such a beautiful act. You can share with the other person what you see in them. You can offer them a window into how they have lifted your soul. And in doing so, maybe you give them just a little more permission to be exactly who they are, appreciate their own strengths, and continue to offer those gifts to many others. Maybe the real reason we don't express our true feelings often enough is because there is something so raw in the act of expressing love for another human being and in allowing yourself to be fully moved by their contribution to you.

When I was growing up, my mom had this amazing habit of sending people written thank you cards. My brother, sister and I used to gently poke fun at her. Before she went to a dinner party, we'd joke, "Mom, have you already written your thank you card?" But now, I realize what a beautiful habit that was.

Following her example, once I was well enough to walk outside and get to a store, I went out and bought a stack of thank you cards. In the mornings, when I was crippled with fatigue and didn't want to get out of bed, the one thing that got me up was remembering that stack of cards and thinking about who I might have the opportunity to thank that day for the contribution they had made to my life. It was such a gorgeous way to start my days. Oh yes, and let's add one more person to my gratitude list: thank you, Mom!

There are a few things I've learned about appreciating others. The first is that it only takes a moment, and doesn't cost anything, so even in our busy lives, we can choose to take this on without much sacrifice!

Second, I've learned that appreciation is more powerful when it's specific. You could easily say: "I love you" or "I appreciate you" and I'm sure that would be received well. However, it's even more touching when you share with someone specifically how they made a difference in your life, in a way that lets them know that you have really seen them. For example: "I appreciate that you checked in on me regularly because it helped me release my worries after a difficult day," or "When you gave me that piece of advice, I took it, and here's how it made a difference for me ..." or even as simple as, "I appreciate that you cooked dinner today, and the potato dish was particularly delicious!" Mostly, it's opening our eyes a little wider to notice the ordinary things that we take for granted; when we allow ourselves to really notice these things, we may realize they're not just ordinary, they're actually quite extraordinary!

The final thing I've learned is that expressing our appreciation for others gets easier with practice. If you're not used to expressing gratitude, it might feel a bit awkward at first. My advice is to not overthink it, and just to do it! You can just start by saying: "I noticed that ..." or "One thing I appreciate about you is ..." and that's all there is to it!

If there is someone you appreciate, why not reach out to them and let them know? It only takes a minute, and it can make such a difference.

Start with strengths

The beautiful thing about cultivating your capacity to appreciate others is that once it becomes a regular practice, you start noticing things that you might have missed before. When I returned back to work, I found that I was much more easily able to notice and appreciate my co-workers for their contributions.

Celebrating others not only creates a more energizing work environment, it also allows you to lean into their strengths. A study by Gallup shows that those who use their strengths every day are six times more likely to be engaged on the job. Many other studies demonstrate how a strengths-based orientation also positively affects happiness, creativity, confidence and growth.

When we see the best in others, they often rise to the occasion. I've seen exceptional teachers, working in disadvantaged communities, who enable students to make remarkable progress, even when so many others had unfairly given up on those kids. Simply by believing in a student's inherent potential, one teacher can transform the trajectory of a child's life. The same can apply for a great boss, parent or friend.

I think the world would look a whole lot different if we built our collectively capacity to see strengths in others. Our day-to-day lives would be so much richer and more fulfilling if more people felt truly seen for their greatest possible selves. And if many more of us were fully unleashed, I bet we'd see an enormous explosion of creativity in the world!

11

Listen generously

Hold space for others

One of my biggest lifelines during this battle was a friend of mine who would reach out to me every day to check in. Even by text message, she was an incredibly good listener. She would follow up on our earlier thread and ask me very specific questions about how I was doing such as, "How did your doctor's appointment go today?" or "Did that new medicine you got yesterday work?" Her acknowledgment of these small details left me with an experience of feeling heard and not alone.

Given how erratic this virus was, I would end each day in a different mood. Some days I would be frustrated, other days I would be scared for the night ahead, and on good days, I might be joyful about a hurdle I had overcome. Having a space every day to share whatever I was feeling with someone who listened well was so important for my healing. It helped me complete my day and have a feeling of release before I went into the difficult nights.

This skill of holding space for others is one that we should all be trained in, as this is a capacity that could transform both our personal and professional relationships. It takes skill to create a safe space where someone feels that they can be fully open. As I think about my friend and others who are good at holding space, I find that they often ask good questions, listen for both what's said and unsaid, pay attention to the deeper emotion or commitment behind what you are sharing, allow you to feel truly heard before offering solutions, keep what you share in confidence, and model vulnerability themselves. I feel incredibly lucky that I have people around me who held space for me as I went through this rollercoaster of a journey. Sometimes, what we need most in difficult times is to be witnessed and heard.

One of the simplest ways to have someone feel heard is simply to play back what they said to you, in a way that has them really know that you have gotten what they shared. I remember sometimes when I was having a really rough day, a friend would say to me, "I'm really sorry you had a hard day," and say it with such genuine empathy that I truly felt like she got what I was going through. Often, simply feeling understood by another person was all I needed to release my anguish from a tough day.

It sounds so basic really that it almost doesn't seem worth saying. Yet if we pay attention to our listening, we'll find that in many of our interactions, we are actually not leaving the other person feeling truly heard. This happens a lot with the people closest to us, especially with our partners and other family members.

When someone says something to us, we might jump right into giving advice, or tell them about our tough day before we've fully acknowledged what they have shared with us about their day, or sometimes we're so distracted that we completely miss that they're even trying to tell us something at all! One of the surest ways to know that you are not hearing someone is if they keep repeating themselves. If that happens, instead of silently blaming them for being a broken record, perhaps it's time to get curious about what they're trying to tell you that you might be missing.

Be aware of your listening filters

While I was lucky to have many people around me who were good listeners, I also experienced what it felt like to *not* be heard, and those encounters were absolutely soul-crushing. In consulting a range of different doctors for my condition, I had some interactions that were extremely challenging. One visit that is etched in my mind is with a doctor who decided early in our interaction that all my symptoms stemmed from anxiety, even though I told him I was suffering from real physical ailments. His exact words were, "Maybe you should try some yoga, honey."

I had been facing disturbing episodes of blurred vision, dizziness and a racing heart, and I knew I needed proper medical support, not patronizing remarks. By the end of the consultation, I felt completely crushed. That same night, my symptoms got so bad that I ended up in the emergency room and had to be pumped with two bags of IV fluids just to get my irregular heart rate steady. Later, it was discovered that many of the symptoms I was dealing with were a result of a lesion that had formed in the frontal lobe of my brain as a result of the virus. Yoga definitely wouldn't have fixed that!

While this interaction and others like it were extremely frustrating, I don't want to put too much blame on doctors, especially not during this pandemic. I know that frontline workers are facing extreme pressure and fatigue, and I have a lot of empathy for what these doctors must be going through, especially in managing an unprecedented patient load in an environment of great uncertainty. At the same time, in the medical world, poor listening and unconscious bias can be dangerous and sometimes even fatal, so it's not something we should readily ignore.

Luckily for me, over the past few months, I did manage to find some doctors who listened well. I remember the first of these visits when one really kind and attentive doctor said to me, "Yes, I've seen others who are going through exactly what you are going through. You're not alone. Don't worry. We may not have all the answers yet, but we are going to do everything we can to help you." After being dismissed by other doctors, this one interaction was so liberating that I nearly wept tears of joy. But it is also frustrating that this level of deep listening is not more widespread.

In our more everyday worlds, so many relationships fall apart because there is an absence of listening, whether at home or in the professional setting. One reason for this is that we have filters that get in the way of our ability to listen and we have not been trained to notice or deal with these. A trap we fall into is presuming to know how someone close to us will react based on how they have reacted in the past. It's funny that we see ourselves as evolving human beings who grow and change over time, but when dealing with other people, we often can't look beyond the fixed caricatures we have of them. We might listen through the filter of "She is always angry" or "He is always dishonest" or "He never gets things done," and then we can't see it any other way.

I'm not saying you shouldn't learn from past experience. However, the minute you put filters into your listening and assume these expectations to be *always* true, you lose your ability to be with another person exactly as they are in that moment.

If you take a minute and explore your own inner monologue about your partner or child or co-worker, I bet you'll start noticing that you listen to them through a filter. What is the persistent story you tell yourself about them? Try letting go of that preconceived notion about them for just one day and see what you discover. I suspect that you might be pleasantly surprised!

Grow our collective listening capacity

There is a much larger systemic issue in our society around how we listen. As the pandemic went on, I was particularly devastated by the news stories about people of color and those on the margins who were being denied the care they needed. Sadly, this wasn't a big surprise. Many studies of the healthcare system have shown that people of color don't get the same level of care as white patients, and that women's real medical concerns are often dismissed as made up, exaggerated, or imagined. When we listen with preconceived notions about certain people, we miss hearing what they are trying to share with us. And it's not just the healthcare system where we see this unconscious bias; unfortunately, these dangerous stereotypes permeate many of our other systems.

In my work in education, I think about what it would look like if we started teaching kids from an early age what it means to actually listen. Listening is such an underdeveloped ability in our world, but if we put our minds to it, we could develop this skill with the same rigor with which we teach subjects like math or science. The irony is that if we want our children to develop their capacity to listen, it will require us as adults to become better listeners as well!

To grow our listening capacities, the first thing we must understand is that the way we see the world may be very different from the way someone else sees the world. We each have a worldview that shapes what we see, but it's so engrained within us, that most of us are not even aware that it exists, or at least are not explicitly aware of it all the time. It's almost as if each of us is wearing a pair of eyeglasses, each with our own unique filter that allows us to see the world in different shades and textures. Yet we walk around believing that everyone else is seeing the exact same world as us. And this is where most misunderstandings begin.

For example, someone who sees the world through a frame that "people cannot be trusted" will have a very different experience of the exact same events than someone who views the world through the frame that "people generally can be trusted." Or someone who views the world through the lens that "your earning potential determines your value in the world" may experience the same set of circumstances very differently from someone whose view is that "hard work and kindness determine your value."

Sadly, the polarization we are seeing in many countries around the world is a signal that we've lost the ability to dialogue with people who see things differently from us. To transform our societies, we must upgrade our capacity to listen to one another. I think the best place to start is close to home within our own families and workplaces. How can we expect our societies to transform if we're not able to transform the quality of listening in our immediate circles?

To get started on this, we must expand our capacity to be open and curious. This seems simple in theory, but we all know it's much more difficult in practice. A couple years back I had an opportunity to practice my listening when I found myself in an hour long-taxi ride and struck up a conversation with the taxi driver. It was clear from the very beginning that we had radically different worldviews. At the time, the country was extremely polarized, and so I had promised myself that the next time I encountered someone with a very different political orientation than me, I would get curious.

After a little dance, the driver and I engaged in conversation. She shared that she was not thrilled about the new immigrants who had moved into her neighborhood. Right away, I felt defensive because my parents are first-generation immigrants, and I started noticing myself making silent judgements about this woman just a few minutes into the ride. However, I had promised myself that I would get curious, and so I tried desperately to interrupt my automatic thoughts, and began to ask her questions: What scared her about these new immigrants? Has she gotten to know any of them? Did she grow up in this community? Soon I learned that she had spent most of her life in one small town, that her family is all still there, and that she had never traveled outside America.

After telling me her story, she started asking about my life. I shared with her that my grandparents are from India, my parents grew up in Africa, and I grew up in Canada. To my surprise, when she heard that my parents were immigrants, she got genuinely curious about their experience. And she confessed that, up until that moment, she hadn't been able to relate much to immigrants because her friends and family had grown up in America. In turn, I acknowl-edged that I might have some preconceived notions myself, particularly about small town America, since I had limited direct exposure to that part of the coun-try. With these honest admissions on the table, we each began to listen to one another with a little more openness. At the end of the ride, as I got out of the taxi, this woman turned to me in a deeply touching moment. She shared that she has a rule never to talk politics with passengers, but that she was surprised by our conversation, and was really glad that we had talked. I felt the same.

What I learned from this experience is that it is possible to engage genuinely with those who have dif-ferent views from us. I'm not saying we have to rush to agreement or give up our values in the process. However, when we listen openly rather than from a view that "they are stupid" or "they just don't get it" or "I have to convince them", we might discover some-thing new. We may still leave disagreeing with one another, but perhaps with a little more appreciation for our shared humanity, despite our differences.

12

Widen your lens

Find a higher vantage point

I once watched a documentary about astronauts reflecting on their experiences of looking back at the Earth for the first time from outer space. One astronaut came to realize that countries and borders didn't really matter so much anymore because ultimately, we are all connected together, and our differences don't look so stark when looking down at the planet from high above. Just like the astronauts who saw something familiar in a whole different light, my experience of battling this illness has been a life-changing one for me. Through it, I have widened my lens on life.

One thing that happens when we step up to a higher vantage point is that we stop worrying so much about little things. Things that worried me just a few months back seem so insignificant now. Just recently, I was doing some Sunday night cooking and I accidentally shattered a glass all over my kitchen floor. When that happened, I surprised myself with my reaction. Instead of getting annoyed, I actually burst out laughing. In the past, something like this would have frustrated me, but this time, I was not the least bit upset. I was just so happy that day to have the energy to be standing, be cooking and be alive!

But we shouldn't wait for a near-death experience to fly to a higher vantage point. Sometimes, simply taking ourselves out of our normal environment can give us a new perspective. In the past, when I was facing a particularly challenging issue at work, I would sit at my desk and focus all my attention on the problem, but sometimes, the more I tried to focus, the more stuck I would get. Now, if I face a tough challenge, I put on my walking shoes and go to the local park; the energy I feel when I'm moving, coupled with a change of scenery, almost always helps me get unblocked.

Other times, we can grow our perspective by putting ourselves in someone else's shoes. This happened for me as I engaged with the COVID-19 online support community. As I read posts from people who were unable to share their diagnosis at work for fear of losing their jobs, my heart cried out for them because I know how lonely this illness can be and cannot imagine the extra burden of having to hide it from others. Hearing their stories reminded me to be grateful for being part of a workplace where I felt so supported by my colleagues—and also just to be able to work at all in a time when so many others were losing their jobs. Having a new vantage point can be an incredible way to gain perspective, and can also be a good reminder not to take things for granted.

Seek multiple perspectives

Another way to widen our lens is to surround ourselves with a diverse set of people who bring different life experiences and perspectives to us. Since all of us hold different lenses for seeing the world, it's good to be able to see things from multiple angles.

When I was battling this virus, I found support in many people who had very different vantage points than me, and each of them helped in vital ways. For example, one friend who had dealt with serious health issues herself gave me useful advice on navigating the healthcare system. Another friend, with expertise in nutrition, coached me on what foods I should and shouldn't be eating to keep my inflammation levels low. My working parent friends helped me feel less guilty about not being able to perform at my pre-COVID levels when they shared that they too were struggling to balance work with their new reality of kids at home.

I am also fortunate to be part of a leadership development community that brings together people from ages 20-90, and it's been incredible to learn together in this intergenerational space. From the older generation, I am reminded to not sweat the small stuff, and to appreciate all the health and mobility I still do have. From the younger age groups, I'm inspired to keep asking bold questions and dream big.

In a time when our social circles are at risk of getting increasingly homogenous, I now feel the opposite pull. I'm inclined now more than ever to grow my circles to include people who have had different experiences than me because there is so much we can learn from those who have walked different paths in life.

So often, we let our social circles be defined for us by circumstance or convenience, but we have the power to create new ones in any moment. It might take a little effort but the people we spend the most time with can radically shape our lives, so why not be more intentional about who is in this circle? Make it a priority to shape it proactively, rather than let it be shaped for you.

Adopt a whole-system view

Another way to shift our perspectives is by building our capacity to see the whole picture. Navigating the healthcare system these past months has reminded me how challenging it can be to take that holistic view, but also why it's so important.

Over the course of my illness, I saw many different doctors, including a pulmonologist, a neurologist, a gastroenterologist, an infectious disease specialist, a cardiologist, and an emergency room physician. Instead of treating me as a whole person, with organs that are interdependent, these specialists mostly addressed my health issues from their own narrow perspectives. It makes total sense given their specialties, so I don't blame them, but as someone who was facing an attack on my entire body, this specialized approach to medicine wasn't really cutting it for me.

At some point, I realized that I needed to take responsibility for seeing the bigger picture because no one else was going to do it. So on flashcards, I wrote up all the abnormal data from my lab work, emergency room visit, and home monitoring data and pasted it on a wall—similar to how detectives map out crimes on TV shows! Soon, I started seeing new patterns, and with this holistic view, I was able to ask better questions of my doctors and take more initiative for my overall recovery.

Soon after, one of my friends encouraged me to find a doctor who practiced integrative medicine. My friend had gone through years of misdiagnosis of an underlying medical condition until she found an integrative doctor who helped her get to a diagnosis that many doctors before had completely missed.

I am so glad I heeded my friend's advice. It was such a relief to finally have a doctor who stopped looking at me as my parts and instead treated me as a whole human being!

One thing the integrative doctor really helped me understand was that we had to get to the underlying root of the problem—my poorly functioning immune system—rather than just tackle the symptoms on the surface. I can tell you that there were days that

I wanted to jump ship and go to a doctor who would give me a quick fix. It would have been far easier to take a sedative to get through restless nights than do the harder, longer work of learning how to build more rest into my day and accept that my healing journey will take time.

As a society, we have become addicted to quick fixes, whether it is fast-acting medicine for a health problem, a sweet treat when we are craving comfort, or a TV binge session when we are feeling bored. The challenge is that if we always go for quick fixes rather than curing what's under the surface, the same problem will keep rearing its ugly head.

I believe that the skill of being able to look at a whole system is something that can be taught and developed. We could be so much more effective at tackling challenges if we all learned to: get curious about the root causes of a challenge rather than focusing on the symptoms; surface multiple viewpoints rather than assuming we hold the whole picture; and work together with others to find solutions rather than trying to do it all on our own. In building these capacities, we can become more creative and resilient in dealing with our challenges.

PART IV

WAKE UP TO WHAT'S POSSIBLE

13

Take a pause

Connect with what really matters

In our always-on culture, we are constantly on the run, often navigating multiple electronic devices, back-to-back meetings, and long to-do lists. Have you ever felt time just disappear, and you're not sure where it went?

Time is something we take for granted. We think we always have more of it until one day, we realize it's finite. In battling this illness, when I felt that my time might be up sooner than I had envisioned, I was jolted wide awake. I started asking myself questions like: What really matters to me? And am I spending my time in line with my deepest intentions?

This virus was essentially a "pause" moment to reflect on my life. It helped me prioritize the relationships and life goals that were most important to me. When I gave myself space to pause, I realized that two things truly mattered to me: connection and contribution.

Many of us have had the conversation about "bucket lists" or the things we would do if we found out we only had months left to live. We imagine that if we had limited time, we might do all the bold and risky things we didn't have the courage to try before. However, on nights when I wondered if I would make it and asked myself these existential questions, the answer was never skydiving or traveling the world. It was much simpler: I would spend time with the people I care about. I wouldn't be distracted while with them. I would give them my full attention. Connection was what mattered.

The other thing I thought about was my purpose. I'm fortunate enough to have a line of work where I have found a sense of meaning. The work I do is about activating human potential by growing a whole new set of leadership capacities in students, teachers, and other leaders around the world who are reimagining education.

I believe that our current education systems are archaic and broken and that it's time for us to imagine something completely different. I'm personally dreaming of schools that help kids discover their own strengths, operate with empathy, work well with others, and become conscientious global citizens. Throughout my illness, I felt motivated to get back to full health so I could return to this work with full energy.

But I also recall times in my life when I wasn't connected to a greater purpose and how demotivating that was. I remember jumping up the corporate ladder while deep down feeling dissatisfied with the way I was spending my days. But it was hard to get off that path because in our always-on culture, we often don't stop for even a minute to question why we are on a hamster wheel. Before we know it, that next promotion is dangling in front of us, and we resign ourselves to our current path, even though, at our core, we long for something different.

Sometimes, when a disorienting event happens in our lives, like the loss of a loved one or a health issue or a milestone birthday, we do pause and ask these bigger questions. But why don't we create room in our lives for these deeper inquiries on a much more regular basis?

While these questions can feel daunting, I can tell you one thing that I have learned: when you think your time is up, your fears begin to seem petty. You start realizing how precious every moment you have is, and you want to be even more intentional about the time you do have. Pausing gives you a chance to break free of all the external forces that try to overwhelm you. When you pause long enough, you might finally let out that inner voice hidden deep inside you that yearns desperately to be heard.

Get to know yourself

I think we've lost the ability to *be with* ourselves. When I was younger, if I was bored or frustrated or angry, I would have no choice but to look inward because there wasn't an immediate distraction around me. However, now most of us have a cell phone that acts almost like an extended limb of our bodies! This means that if something goes wrong, stopping to inquire into what's actually happening inside us takes enormous discipline— a discipline that we have not cultivated. And so, I'd assert, that most of barely know ourselves, or at least, not at the depth that's possible.

A consequence of this is that we walk around overwhelmed, tired and reactive to the world around us. We take on so many things in our lives, not because we deeply desire them, but because we have been socially conditioned to follow a certain path. Most of us have never bothered to know ourselves deeply enough to imagine what we really want.

In those rare moments that we do look inward, if we sense discomfort, we run away, rather than looking deeper. We have been taught discomfort is a bad thing and must immediately be squelched, so most of us don't know what to do with it when it arises, other than to run from it or numb it.

It's such a shame that we've lost this ability to pause and be with ourselves because I believe there is incredible wisdom within each one of us. So how can we tap into this? One way to start is to simply give yourself a few minutes every day to connect with your deepest self. You could ask yourself a daily question like: What matters to me? What's alive in me right now? What do I feel most called to do today?

Over time, if we get to know ourselves more deeply, we'll learn to tap into this intuition when making choices, whether it's big life decisions or the series of everyday micro-decisions that, when added together, are actually the ones that shape our lives.

Build a pause practice

I have found that having a regular reflective practice is absolutely essential not just to know yourself, but also to ensure that your energy aligns with your intentions.

Over the years, I have developed a weekly practice that has kept me grounded. Every Sunday, I take a few moments to reflect on the past week and get clear on my intentions for the week ahead. This practice turned out to be very useful when I fell ill.

After a few days of being sick, I decided to keep a daily journal to track how I was doing. Each day, I would jot down a few notes to capture the day—what medicines I had taken, how I was feeling, how much sleep I got, and anything else that was notable about that day. Then on Sundays, I would go back through that journal and reflect on the past week to see where I had made progress, where I had gotten stuck, and what that might mean for the following week. In these Sunday reflection sessions, I often made important discoveries.

For example, as I ended week five of this illness, I reviewed my daily journal and realized that I had made huge progress on most symptoms except for one. For the past weeks, I had been suffering from terrible insomnia and was getting only 2-4 hours of sleep each night. I was pretty much a walking zombie, and it wasn't pretty! So in line with my biggest intention—to get back into good health—my week six intention was to find a path to getting more sleep. When I was able to focus my energy on a specific challenge, I found that I had a greater chance of breaking through.

While a weekly reflective practice is a powerful way to notice things that are holding you back, you don't always have to focus on problems. In fact, a few months into my daily journaling practice, I realized that I was getting weary because writing down all the ways my body was failing me suddenly felt very heavy. And the last thing I needed at the end of a long, hard day was anything that further sapped my energy. To spice things up a little, I decided to add a new prompt to reflect on each day: "What brought me joy today?" It was a simple question but in it I discovered so much!

I discovered that my daily walks brought me tremendous delight. Or that when I had a strong start to the morning, it put me in a good mood for the rest of the day. In just asking myself this one additional question, my daily 2-minute journaling exercise began bringing a smile to my face and also inspired me to keep up with the good stuff. For example, discovering that my daily walk was consistently one of my bright spots each day helped me stay committed to that habit, even when I felt fatigued or when the weather turned cold. My walking habit soon became an unshakeable ritual!

A powerful question that you ask yourself regularly is one of the greatest reflective tools. This past year, I focused on: What were my accomplishments and disappointments this past week? What's bringing me joy? And what will I try newly next week? However, you can choose any question you want depending on what's most important for you to reflect on. I have a friend who picks a word or phrase for the year, such as "Energetic" or "The Year of Yes", and then every week reflects on how she's doing with that intention.

Building a reflective practice seems simple, but I'll have to admit that in times of extreme stress, it can be easy to rush into the day without making space for this. I think it's because every aspect of our culture has been designed to prioritize the urgent over the important. And yet it's precisely the times when we are busiest or most stressed that we need these reflective practices the most.

The best way to start a regular reflective practice is to set aside just a few minutes a day, ideally keeping it small and manageable at first until you build it into a habit. If you can tie it to your morning coffee routine, or your evening commute, or some other regular daily event, you may have a better chance of sticking with it!

One of the most common excuses for not having a regular reflective ritual is, "I don't have time for this." The irony is that a regular pause practice actually creates more time in your life because you are likely to discover better and faster approaches to dealing with persistent challenges! You'll also likely find much greater peace of mind as you clear away all the things that have being weighing on you subconsciously.

Take a collective pause

So often our lives are on autopilot, but moments of crisis force us to pause and ask more existential questions. At the most fundamental level, our first inquiry in times of crisis should be: What are the most important questions we should be asking ourselves at this time?

One pressing question on my mind these days is: How do we create a world that is more equitable? I think about this question daily in my own work, as I see the existing inequities in the world being further magnified by this pandemic. In my work at Teach For All, I support a network of leaders around the world who are working to ensure that all children, especially those coming from the most vulnerable communities, have the opportunity to fulfil their potential. Despite my own ordeal, I am acutely aware of my privilege and know that many people are struggling under far worse circumstances than I am.

For those living in slum communities, social distancing is not a possibility. For those without health insurance, basic medicines are not available. For those who have lost their livelihood, it may be a struggle to pay their rent. For those facing domestic violence, my solitary living environment would probably seem like a welcome relief. For children around the world who rely on school for free meals, school closures have also meant hunger. A question I am asking myself now is, *How can we use this moment to reimagine our systems and address these inequities?*

Soon after this pandemic hit, we also faced a growing recognition of racial injustice in America. For days, protestors marched down my street, outraged at the killing of yet another unarmed black man symbolizing centuries of systemic racial injustice. These inequities have always existed, but the conversation about them can no longer be limited to the victims of these inequities. It's time to wake up, have these conversations at a much wider level, and act. In this moment, when there is so much suffering and upheaval all at once, I hope we begin to ask the questions that really matter: What would it look like to treat every human being with dignity? What must we fundamentally transform in ourselves and in the way we relate to one another?

A related question on my mind is how we define success in our society. So many of the success stories flaunted by the media are of business tycoons, athletes, and other celebrities. We worship the individual "hero" leader. Yet, when we look at what really makes up the fabric of our society, what about the everyday heroes who contribute to the greater good?

Clapping for frontline workers or others in service isn't enough. We need to renegotiate social contracts. This demands a much larger conversation and requires asking difficult questions about power dynamics in our society. I keep wondering why we call these workers "essential" but pay them so little. Why is it that we celebrate philanthropists who give money but rarely value the nurses and teachers who give their time? What could our world look like if we ended our obsession with a "me" culture and instead truly valued those who serve? I only hope we pause long enough to make sure that we're asking ourselves the right questions at this turning point for our collective humanity.

14

Acknowledge death

How do you want to leave?

Why is it that we are so afraid to talk about death in Western cultures? More than once on this harrowing journey I felt my time was up, and I was forced to contemplate death.

The biggest pang I felt when I let myself consider this prospect was all the people I would leave behind. Nine years ago, my 46-year-old uncle died suddenly of a heart attack, and I travelled to Mexico for his funeral. Given how young and seemingly healthy he was, he did not have all of his end-of-life affairs in order, and so adding to the pain of his loss was the chaos that ensued as we tried to figure out these other details. This worry about causing my loved ones any more pain than was absolutely necessary prompted me to sit down one day and write my will, during a moment when I had some uncertainty about how this all might end.

These logistical acts and ensuing conversations with loved ones can be difficult because they're not the norm, especially for younger people. But I have learned that the best way to embrace such challenges is simply to buck up and take the first step. After I wrote my will, I called my mother and sister and had a conversation with them about it. It was a little awkward, of course, but we got through it. It even prompted my family members to contemplate these same questions for themselves.

Another question that came up for me was what I would want others to do if I ever got to the point where I could not make a decision for myself. As I speak frankly with my friends who are doctors, they often lament how, in Western societies in particular, we expend so much energy on extending the last days of peoples' lives, without duly considering the consequences of this approach. I got clear for myself what I would want in this situation, and I think it's an important question for all of us to consider.

On a more personal note, I watched my grandfather's journey before he passed away. When he was healthy, I remember him being so disciplined about his daily walks and getting dressed with such care. Yet in his final months, when these simple routines were not manageable for him anymore, I wondered if he was hanging on not for himself but for all of us who surrounded him. It makes me think about the quality of life that so many face in their final days. What if we didn't shy away from this conversation about death and talked more openly about what it means to live and let go with grace?

How do you want to live?

While I expected the prospect of death would be scary, I soon discovered that I was not so much afraid of dying. If anything, my fear was of not having fully lived. Luckily, as my life flashed before my eyes during those contemplative moments, I came to the realization that I have indeed lived! I have loved with reckless abandon and experienced so much joy in my life. I have travelled to distant places and met amazing people from all around the world. I have laughed until my belly hurts. I have made ample time for family and friends. I have hobbies that bring fun into my life. I have discovered work that gives me purpose. All in all, I have had the good fortune of living a life rich with love and laughter.

My biggest regret, if you can call it that, is that at 40 years old, I am only now finally finding my voice. I'm ready to create. I'm ready to make a contribution. I feel like I've taken a lot from the world in the first stretch of my life, and now I am ready to give back. I yearn to hang on a little longer so I can take all the blessings that life has thrown my way and commit to something much bigger than myself from this point forward.

A final epiphany I had as I contemplated my life was wondering not about what I had accomplished in my life, but about who I had been along the way. Had I been kind to my family and friends? Had I taken full responsibility for my mistakes? Had I expressed myself fully and let the world see who I really am? We spend so much of our lives focused on what we are doing, but when the end feels near, perhaps all that matters is who we are being.

In our materialistic world, much of the focus of life is on *doing*. But does that really matter? What use are all the accomplishments in the world if you've been a jerk to others in getting there? Sure, maybe the outside world might give you some applause, but deep inside, I imagine it's a terribly lonely place.

The other challenge with a focus on "doing" is that while we are obsessed with the chase to get to the next milestone, it's a never-ending race; once you get what you want, you immediately want more. You might get a promotion at work, and before you have a chance to truly celebrate that, you're already thinking about the next rung on the ladder. Or you might find yourself a small apartment only to start dreaming about the bigger house. Or you might get engaged to someone, only to start thinking about the wedding, and then when you will have kids. This approach to living is not wrong. It just focuses our attention on the future and on the external world around us.

There is another way to think about life, and that is to focus on who we are *being* in the present moment. Are we being generous, joyful, free, courageous, playful, and alive? Are we even aware of our states of being? I feel that in today's society, we measure so much of our success by what we are "doing" that we have forgotten how much of life comes from who we are "being."

The irony is that if we could focus on being these things *now*, then maybe our obsession with chasing the next milestone wouldn't feel as pressing. Instead of waiting for the next promotion or the next step in our relationship to feel joyful or free, we could just be that way *now*!

I have found that a simple way to bring more of a "being" paradigm into your life is to pick a word or two to define how you want to live your life. Do you want your life to be about courage, service, generosity, or something else? I won't lie. Once you're intentional about this, you will likely have a lifelong journey of aligning your actions to those intentions. A true test of whether you're "being" in line with who you say you are is if these are the words others would immediately use to describe you without being prompted. So perhaps a first inquiry question is, *What are the words you would want others to shout out if asked about you?*

Death is an inevitable fate that we will all face someday. Instead of being intimidated by it, we can use it as a guiding force to live purposefully with the time we do have.

15

Stand out rather than fit in

Stand out

A favorite quote of mine comes from the children's book author Dr. Seuss: *"Why fit in when you were born to stand out?"* We spend our lives longing to belong, but when you think your time is up, fitting in seems so irrelevant—and frankly, a little boring! Instead, you begin to wonder whether you expressed your ideas fully, offered your unique gifts to the world, and took enough risks. You have an urge to be a creative force in service of something much bigger than yourself, something that might last beyond you when your time is up.

As I struggled with this illness, I was lucky to benefit from many wise people who were not afraid to stand out. As one example, I was grateful for Chris Cuomo, a CNN journalist, who had the guts to express himself openly about his battle with this virus when so little was still known about it. When I fell ill, it was still the very early days of the pandemic so I didn't personally know others who had faced COVID-19. However, every night at 9 p.m., Chris Cuomo would report from his basement about his own battle with the virus because he was committed to helping others learn more about something that was so opaque to us all at that time. When I started facing crazy symptoms like night hallucinations, I felt a little less alone knowing that someone else had also experienced "the beast" and had come out alive at the other end!

So often, we put a shield up in front of us rather than expressing ourselves fully. We sacrifice what makes us special in the name of belonging. We're so afraid to look silly or be laughed at that we hide a piece of ourselves. The sad part is that we weren't born that way. I have several nieces and nephews, and I have loved watching them in the toddler stage. Toddlers are incredibly expressive beings because they're not afraid to look silly. They don't even have that chip active in their brains yet. Yet at some point in our childhoods, most of us go through an embarrassing or difficult moment that unwittingly kills off some of our natural playful energy from that point onward.

I remember one such incident when I was six years old. I was running down the school hallway toward my best friend, with a bundle of energy because it was morning recess and time to go outside! As I roared down the hallway, I accidentally bumped into my friend. The teacher scolded me indoors while all the kids went out to play for the break.

At lunch time, when I finally went outside, my so-called best friend and another girl stood on top of a hill in the playground and laughed at me. And in that moment, a little piece of the free-spirited, risk-taking Radha died, and I became slightly more cautious, and a little more wary of other peoples' laughter.

It sounds kind of ridiculous now, but we all have these incidents when we were expressing ourselves in the world, and then something happened that stifled this. And whether we know it or not, these incidents subconsciously stay with us, and limit our ability to fully express ourselves in the world.

So instead of standing out, we focus on belonging, because we're afraid to be exposed again. The real shame is that, it's not just our weaknesses or insecurities that we hide, but also the wonderful things about us that make us special. In that uniqueness, there is so much beauty, yet many of us shy away from letting the world really see us. And what a shame this is! It relegates us to being ordinary when we could instead be extraordinary. Imagine a world where the greatest poets, musicians, scientists, writers or entrepreneurs had held back from expressing themselves fully in the world. Our world would be so dull!

The reality is that there is greatness in all of us, but somewhere between childhood and growing up, we forget that. What was it that you loved doing as a child, and what if you discovered that again? Where are you holding yourself back or hiding for the sake of belonging, and what might be possible if you gave yourself permission to stand out?

Stop being afraid and just do it

There is an obsession in our society with "getting it right." Instead of dreaming and acting big, many of us stop ourselves from pursuing great ideas because we lack confidence or aim for too much perfection.

Courage requires letting go of the desire to look good, or the fear of looking bad. It appears when we stop being afraid. And through this experience, I started wondering, why do I get afraid, anyway? In the past months, I had several moments when I truly feared for my life. But in my regular day-to-day existence, it's not like there is a real danger to my life in most pursuits I take on. So why live in fear? What's the worst that can happen?

As an example, at 3 a.m. one night when I was facing a bout of insomnia, I had a random thought to write this very book. Then almost immediately, my inner monologue kicked in: *That's ridiculous. Who am I to write anything? What do I even have to say anyway?* Under ordinary circumstances, I might have just stopped right there. But in that moment, I realized I had absolutely nothing left to lose. I didn't want to wait until tomorrow or the next week. Given the unpredictability of this virus, I couldn't be sure that I'd still be here. So that night, I got up and started writing. And I wrote and wrote and wrote. And 24 hours later, I had 50 pages and 10 chapters written.

Once I finished, I had another choice. I could just keep this private or do something with it. Again, my inner monologue started: *This is not ready to share. You* *wrote it in 24 hours while in an incapacitated mental state. You probably have more work to do before it's ready for primetime.* Typically, I might have just held on to it and tried to "get it right" before sharing, but this time I said to myself: "F*&k it! What's the worst that can happen anyway? No one reads it. People don't like it. So what? At least it occupied my mind on one restless night and helped me process this difficult time. And in taking it on, I dared to try something new!" A minute later, I opened my phone, hit send, and shared it with a friend.

And I felt liberated. Even if this was a complete failure, I didn't really care that much anymore. What mattered more was that I put myself out there.

I've always admired people around me who I experience as courageous. It's something I want to grow more in myself. As I was reflecting on what courage means for me, I realized that some of my proudest moments in life have been when I put myself out there or said and did something in line with my values even if it was not popular. Even if I later suffered some external consequences for my words or actions, at least I had some inner peace knowing that I didn't hold back when it mattered.

Failure is only failure because we tie so much of our self-worth to extrinsic measures of value, such as fame, money and public acknowledgment. However, if we start judging things more by intrinsic factors, like learning, growth, and self-expression, then maybe we never really fail at all so long as we have enough reflective muscle in us to learn from every experience.

I think being brave just takes practice. The more you get clear on what's important to you and the more you stand for this, the more you realize that you are not going to die from things that seem to terrify you. You might as well keep putting yourself out there, stand for something, and live a little!

For me, I'm emerging from all of this willing to take more risks. This experience has given me a sense of urgency. When I have an idea or feel called to do something, I am no longer going to wait for someday. All we have for certain is *right now*.

Create a non-conformist world

Thinking even bigger, what would the world look like if every one of us felt fully free to express ourselves in the world? And what if our education systems were designed so that children were encouraged to discover and express the beautiful unique gifts that each of them possesses inside? With so many kids out of school or being forced to learn in new ways, this feels like a perfectly ripe moment to reimagine education and ask ourselves the most fundamental questions: Why do we educate? What is the ultimate purpose of education? What if schools were a place where kids could truly discover their full self-expression, creativity, and purpose? What if kids were rewarded for standing out rather than fitting in?

I also believe that courage is a mindset we can proactively grow in children. As a woman in the field of education, I think especially about how we can cultivate this orientation in young girls. Girls often have brilliant and creative ideas, but don't always feel brave enough or supported enough to express them. So how do we break this cycle early? We need to use all the tools at our disposal—education, media, and parenting—to encourage all children to believe in themselves and put forward their ideas into the world. And we need to de-stigmatize failure and help children see mistakes as an integral part of learning rather than as a source of shame.

Since children learn a tremendous amount from watching the adults around them, all of us who spend time with kids could benefit from gently interrogating our own relationship to failure and belonging. I bet children would learn a lot more from us if we adults got braver in expressing our truest selves!

16

Create your life

Let go of "should"

A few years ago, I started to learn how to surf. What I discovered about the ocean is that it's unpredictable. You ride up and down with the waves, but you never really know which wave is going to carry you to shore or which one might pummel you unexpectedly. The ocean can be calm one moment, and then things can turn with a sudden gust of wind.

Just like the ocean, we operate in living systems that are ever-changing and dynamic, but we fool ourselves into thinking that there is a straight, predictable path. We have this false notion that life "should be" a particular way, that there is one endpoint and a clear path to get there.

We also have these fixed, and often unconscious, notions of ourselves—that we are a particular way, and that's the way we'll always be, and that these traits define us in all circumstances. For example, I might think of myself as adventurous, active, hard-working, introverted, or disorganized. But in creating these labels, I limit myself to a fixed identity and don't give myself room to grow.

I had an epiphany around all of this one day on my daily walk to the park as I passed by the tennis courts where I used to play. My doctor told had me that except for walking, I wasn't allowed to exercise anymore. As someone who had been extremely active before, this new constraint felt very tough. Every time I walked by those tennis courts, I would get a pang in my stomach and think to myself: "I am 40 years old and have taken good care of myself. I should be sprinting around those courts right now!" For me, that's the way life "should" have been.

Finally, after months of that angst-ridden walk, it suddenly hit me. I had been clinging on to a definition of how life *should be*—that at 40 years old, I "should" be in perfect health with no limitations. With that as my frame for how life should be, no wonder I felt disappointed every day. At that moment, I realized that unless I shifted my outlook, I would spend my life constantly feeling inadequate given my current physical state. I decided to let go of this "ideal picture" of how life should be and just embrace reality. The fact was that I was able to walk. The fact was also that I was unable to sprint. That's all there was to it. This was my truth at that moment.

Many ideas about the way life should be are imposed on us by society. We *should* get married by a certain age. We *should* stay with our partners for a lifetime. We *should* hit certain milestones in our career at the same time as our peers. We *should* always be in perfect health. Then life hits us with curveballs and we struggle because we are comparing our actual lives to this ideal version of what our lives should be. But what if we let go of the idea that life "should" be some particular way? We'll still face life's waves, but we can be much more at peace as we ride through them.

It's incredible how easily we fall prey to the "should" trap. I chuckled at myself several times while writing this book because I would catch myself saying I "should" have finished this book earlier and got it out quicker. It's ironic that even when I'm writing about "should" behavior, I'm succumbing to it! After I had a little laugh at myself, I was able to let go of my own "should" thinking around the timing of this book; once I did, I had a lot more fun finishing the last pieces. It's amazing how much lighter life can be when we let go of "shoulds!"

Dare to create

When we were kids, we dreamed. Our imaginations ran wild. We made up make-believe lands. But somewhere along the journey to adulthood, we stopped playing, and along the way, we also stopped dreaming.

In these past months, I have given myself space to pause and dream again. I started asking myself questions like: What do I really want in life? What do I long for? What are my biggest boldest dreams? If I had no constraints, what would I jump into headfirst?

I'll admit that at first, I wasn't that good at dreaming. Most of us aren't, because we haven't truly exercised this muscle for a long time. My initial dreams were nice, but a little conventional or just an incremental improvement over my current reality.

So I kept digging and allowed myself to dream bigger. I began dreaming of relocating to a place where I could wake up near the ocean every day. I dreamt of an education system where all children had a safe, trusting, loving space to flourish, and where we teach our kids how to listen, how to be compassionate, and how to express their true beauty in the world. I dreamt of a world where we focus more on what's working and what's good about people rather than on what's not working and what's wrong with people. And I found myself smiling as I connected with what truly lit me up.

What is the big bold dream that you have deep inside you? What if just for a moment you parked all the reasons and excuses that get in the way of that dream? What might be possible if you allowed yourself to explore with playfulness and curiosity?

Too often, we stop ourselves from dreaming because we get caught up in all the reasons those dreams are not possible—maybe it's financial constraints, or family obligations, or other responsibilities. Sure, we can't magically wish all these constraints away.

However, if we're really honest with ourselves, we'll likely discover that, some of the reasons that stop us from pursuing our dreams could be surmounted, if we allowed ourselves to really take a look. The challenge is that we rarely dig deep enough to explore this space because it forces us to confront things that scare us. What if I tell my loved ones about my dreams and they laugh at me? What if I put my heart and soul into something I really care about, and it fails? And maybe most powerful: *What if I go for it and it is everything I have ever hoped for?*

Yes, these things can seem daunting, and so it's easy to retreat to comfort, familiarity and safety. However, what we sacrifice when we suppress our deepest dreams and desires is the freedom, joy and adventure that can awaken from a life truly fulfilled.

The sad part is that most of us accept the norms we inherited from our upbringing and from society at large, without really allowing ourselves to imagine what else might be possible. I'll be honest that for the first three decades of my life, I followed milestones that were expected of me, without really questioning them fully.

Allowing ourselves to explore alternate paths takes some resolve because we have to stop hiding behind all the reasons and excuses that hold us back. It's scary to take a leap and pursue big uncertain dreams rather settle for something mediocre. But it's also incredibly freeing when we finally get that we have way more power than we admit to be designers of our own lives.

What I am clear about now is that our time on this planet is very short. I for one don't want to be reactive and let life happen to me. I don't want to be a bystander in my life. I don't want to end my life with a boatload of regrets. I want to create my life.

PART V

LIVE BEYOND YOU

17

Practice compassion

Start with self-compassion

When we think about compassion, we think about turning our attention to others. Yet in order to be compassionate with others, I believe that we must start with ourselves. We are really much too hard on ourselves, and this leads us to be hard on other people as well.

I know for certain that I was critical of myself many times throughout this journey, especially on days when I felt like I wasn't recovering fast enough.

Many days I would start my day with energy, but by about 10 a.m., my body would get so fatigued that I would need to lie down. When I lay down, though, my mind was not at ease. Silently, I would be judging myself for not being able to break through this illness.

Finally, I realized that this approach just wasn't working. This angst was miserable, and definitely not good for my recovery! What's more, others around me were being much kinder to me than I was being to myself. I finally had a breakthrough on all this when I asked myself, "What advice would I give to a friend in a similar situation?" It was easy. I would tell them, "Give yourself some grace and be gentle with yourself." And so I had to start taking my own advice!

We all have things we don't like about ourselves, and we say these to ourselves all the time. *I'm not smart enough. I'm not productive enough. I'm not attractive enough. I am not liked enough. I am not good enough.* It can go on and on. We spend our whole lives silently judging ourselves. Or trying to fix ourselves.

What if, instead of trying to fix ourselves, we accepted these imperfect parts of ourselves as absolutely perfect, as an expression of being human—beautiful and flawed all at the same time—just like every other human being?

When I started accepting my imperfections, it was quite freeing, and I also started feeling more connected with others. For example, on days when I felt that I was not productive enough, it helped to know that many other people around the world felt the same way.

As we begin to accept our own imperfections, two things become possible in our relationship with others. First, when we can accept ourselves, we grow our capacity to accept imperfections in others. Second, when we are feeling more secure with ourselves, we are less likely to project our insecurities on others.

Get in other people's worlds

Once you have compassion for yourself, you're able to be much more compassionate with others. This is especially important in times of collective trauma when everyone seems to be operating from heightened triggered states. It's a dangerous place to be in when instead of compassion talking to compassion, triggers are talking to triggers.

I faced a situation like this the first time I called 911. The day I made the call, I was terrified. My blood pressure had dropped suddenly, I felt dizzy and everything suddenly went blurry. When the paramedics arrived on scene, one of them was in a raging mood. He was ranting so angrily that even his partner told him to calm down. I felt intimidated by his anger. Here I was in my most vulnerable state, and his rage made me feel less safe to ask questions and seek help. The next day, I realized I felt very angry at him in return.

But a few days later, in the news, I read about a medical professional who had been so overwhelmed by the stress of the pandemic, that she finally took her own life. At that moment, I got it. Just like me, the paramedic was scared. Just like me, he was angry at what was happening in the world. In the simple act of entering my home, this man was putting himself at risk of infection. I softened a lot when I realized that, underneath our fierce exteriors, we likely had something in common: we were both just terrified.

After this incident, I recommitted to a practice I had learned years ago called metta (or loving kindness) meditation. It's a simple practice that I do every evening now for 10 minutes. In the practice, you visualize certain people and then offer them loving and kind thoughts for a moment or two. First, you start with yourself. Then a good friend or family member for whom you have positive feelings. Then a stranger. And then someone for whom you might have negative feelings that day. Sometimes I use a simple phrase as I hold others in my thoughts such as, "May they be healthy, may they be happy, may they live with ease." I find that this practice softens me up and allows me to find compassion for others, even those who I might have felt anger or frustration toward just a few minutes before.

I remember one week when someone in my life had really irritated me. The first time I thought of him in my evening loving-kindness practice, I tried to have positive thoughts and completely failed. At that moment, I had a fleeting thought that maybe this practice is a farce and doesn't really work for *all* people. Thankfully though, I decided to keep at it. For the following few nights, for just a couple of minutes, I would hold this person in my thoughts. After five days of doing this, something finally shifted. While I was trying to cling on to my anger for dear life, at some point, I just couldn't anymore! I had initially painted a story of this guy as a villain, and now all I could see was that he was probably going through a difficult time himself, and I just couldn't help but feel some warmth toward him. The next time I interacted with him, everything felt a lot lighter, like a load had finally been lifted.

The truth is that we can't control the external world around us, even though many of us would love to have that superpower. We try so hard to fix the people in our lives and assume they're the unruly ones, not us. Or we attempt to micro-manage situations to feel some semblance of control in a world brimming with uncertainty. But trying to fully control people or external circumstances around us rarely works. What we do have power over is our inner world, and the perspective we choose to bring to every situation. Once we begin to accept this, everything changes. We start to see that by simply altering how we view people, we can transform the quality of our relationships. And by transforming the quality of our relationships, we can transform the quality of our lives.

18

Be a contribution

Embrace interconnectedness

When we focus too much on ourselves, it robs us of joy. In Western societies, in particular, we walk around thinking about ourselves as separate from others. We spend much of our time trying to defend ourselves, be right about our opinions, or avoid being controlled by others. In this version of the world, we are "over here," and the other person is "over there," and there is a massive barrier in between us.

The reality though is that we are not so separate. In South Africa, there is an idea known as *Ubuntu,* which essentially means: "I am because you are." It implies that we do not exist in such isolation and that our humanity is intricately tied up in each other. So many other ancient traditions emphasize this same idea—that we are deeply and profoundly interconnected as human beings and with all living things.

At a societal level, I fear that we're facing a real crisis in connection in that we've lost our ability to interact with those who are different from us. When we "other" people, we forget something fundamental: that we are all interconnected, and that ultimately, our fates are intertwined.

The civil rights activist Martin Luther King Jr. put this so beautifully when he said: *"We are all caught in an inescapable network of mutuality, tied in a single garment of destiny. And what affects one directly affects all indirectly. For some strange reason, I can never be what I ought to be until you are what you ought to be. And you can never be what you ought to be until I am what I ought to be."*

This network of mutuality also exists at a more personal level in almost every moment of our daily lives. Just imagine walking into your living room and realizing that your loved one is angry with you. Their anger likely triggers something in you, and all of a sudden, you find yourself angry as well.

Now imagine a different scenario. You walk into the room, and your loved one is radiating with joy. That also can shift something in you, but in a very different way.

This notion that one person's fate is intertwined with one another's means that we have an incredible responsibility for how we "show up" every day. Each of us has the power to shift things around us simply by how we are being around others. Since we're all interconnected like a spider web, one act of kindness can spread kindness, while one act of anger can spread anger. The question each of us must ask ourselves is: *What chain reaction do we personally want to set into motion?*

While the pandemic led to some isolation, paradoxically, it also fostered connection in new ways. I, for one, discovered incredible joy and aliveness in being interdependent with others over this past year. Like many during the pandemic, because of social distancing rules, my social circles this year shrank to a small handful of people, but with those people, I found myself engaging much more deeply than ever before.

Something about choosing a core set of people to hunker down with got me wondering about these relationships. Why is it that I choose to spend my time with these people? And why is it that they choose to spend their time with me?

I realized that there were two types of bonds that really flourished for me. First, I found myself strengthening connections with my immediate family and with a few solid long-term friends who had been fixtures in my life for a while. In these relationships, we offered each other security and comfort. Having a stable presence gave all of us some much-needed groundedness in an otherwise tumultuous environment.

In addition to these long-standing relationships, I also developed a couple of new deep friendships through this rocky year. What I got from those was different. The presence of new energy brought me inspiration and a sense of adventure, which was very much welcomed in a year when day-to-day life felt a little mundane. In these newer relationships, I was not constrained by a fixed identity or expectations that, often subconsciously, come with long-standing relationships; I had the chance to play a little, and discover and express myself in new ways. It was so freeing to have a new space to evolve and grow, especially as the world around me changed so rapidly.

I came to truly appreciate both these types of relationships—old and new—for together, they gave me ground to stand on, and room to fly. Thanks to this deeply fulfilling set of relationships, I experienced a surprising amount of joy in a year that was otherwise filled with challenges and uncertainty.

Through our deepest relationships, we get to discover who we are in the world. We learn what we're capable of offering others, and we also get to grow from their contributions to us. Ultimately, the most beautiful relationships are a playful dance, where the magic comes not from who we are being as individuals, but who we get to be when we are together.

Commit to something bigger than you

One of the things I found hardest about this illness was that, during my recovery, I needed to focus a lot of attention on myself. It makes sense rationally. I had limited energy and needed to direct it wisely toward my own healing. Yet this focus on myself felt so empty at times, especially when the world felt like it was on fire and so many other people around me needed support and care.

Once I gained some strength back, I went back into the online communities that had been a source of comfort for me, and began responding to messages there. Sometimes it would be as simple as responding to a newcomer who had just tested positive for the virus, letting them know that they were not alone. Mostly, I was hoping that I could ease someone else's pain just a little, as so many others had done for me.

The more time I spent in these groups though, the more I was blown away by the incredible care that complete strangers in these groups were offering one another. Some community members would share detailed posts about treatments they were trying so that others could have better questions to ask their own doctors. Others would offer words of solidarity to those feeling isolated, including many who were the only ones in their families or workplaces with this virus. I experienced so much warmth in these spaces that it gave me a deep faith in the beauty of humanity even during my darkest hours.

The irony is that it's in these moments when we give to others, rather than the ones when we're focused on ourselves, that we feel most at peace. Our individualistic societies are built around a false premise that securing more for yourself is the source of happiness. Yet I have found quite the opposite to be true. When we're able to contribute to others, even in small ways, we don't have to chase happiness anymore; it emerges naturally.

There is something quite innate about this relationship between giving and happiness because these tendencies start at a very young age. In one study, toddlers under 2 years old were given goldfish crackers and asked to give away one of their crackers to someone else. Researchers evaluated the toddlers' facial expressions and found that they exhibited greater happiness when they gave away their treats versus when they received treats for themselves.[8]

During my recovery, I was the recipient of so many gestures of kindness from others. I was grateful for each act of compassion, whether it was a thoughtful gift or a loving text message.

I was so moved by these small acts of kindness from others, that it reminded me how I could also be there for others. One day, a doctor friend of mine had endured a particularly rough shift in a hospital environment that sounded like a war zone. To lighten up her day, I sent her an Amazon gift certificate to buy baking supplies since I knew that conjuring up chocolate treats was her form of release at the end of a gruelling week. There is something so healing in turning your attention to others. In those instances when I was able to turn outward, I momentarily forgot about my own issues.

I believe that every one of us is capable of living a life of service. When it comes from a genuine place, rather than from a sense of obligation, a life of service is so much more enriching and fulfilling than a life of selfishness. Service can look very different for different people. Some may serve by being parents or caregivers. Some might pursue service vocations such as teaching or medicine. A taxi driver or hairdresser may choose to serve others by offering a kind listening ear. What service looks like can vary from person to person, but the reality is that every one of us has something to give. This opens some beautiful life-long questions that each of us might ponder: What unique gifts do I have to offer to others? And who am I—or who could I be—as a contribution in this world?

(Full disclosure: my Amazon baking goods gift to my friend might have been a bit selfish, as I have since received many batches of delicious homemade fudge!)

Activate our collective power

Many nights I thought about what might be possible if we disrupted the dominant paradigm of individualism prevalent in so many Western societies and started embracing our collective spirit. In many places in the world, there has been a gradual erosion of communal culture and civil society. We are now seeing the dire consequences of that self-oriented way of living.

For starters, many people are miserable in their day-to-day living. A Gallup worldwide poll shows that only 15% of workers feel engaged at work. In civil society, we see massive divisions arising, with people unable to converse anymore with those who hold opposing political views. And our earth is suffering as we act as if the planet we live on is separate from ourselves and can handle all our abuse. All these effects are outcomes of an overemphasis on a "me" rather than a "we" culture.

However, it doesn't have to be this way. During the early days of the virus' outbreak, I saw so many beautiful examples of local communities coming together to support one another. As one example, when the pandemic first struck New York, there was a shortage of medical equipment in New York hospitals, so someone in my apartment building organized a group of people to 3-D print masks for the local hospital. In another instance, several young residents in my building offered to do grocery runs for their at-risk elderly neighbors who were afraid to venture out themselves.

In my workplace, I also saw countless examples of communities coming together at a global level to tackle common challenges. Soon after the pandemic unfolded, hundreds of teachers in communities around the world came together on a WhatsApp group, now known as the Teaching Without Internet Alliance, to share ideas for how to support student learning during school closures in contexts where kids didn't have internet access at home. It was incredible to see teachers from Chile to Nigeria using low bandwidth tools such as WhatsApp and public radio to reach kids in hard-to-reach communities, and even more incredible to see how all of these teachers then came together as a larger global community to share what they were learning, in a true expression of camaraderie and creativity!

As we decide how to lead in this era, I hope we can move away from the adulation of individual hero leaders, and instead elevate the idea of collective leadership. The challenges we face in our society are so complex that no one single person holds the answer. When I think about the biggest societal challenges of our time, real change will need to come ground up from communities, rather than top down.

The sad part is that, over the past decades, we've lost a lot of our sense of community, though perhaps the silver lining of this pandemic is that it's enabling this collective spirit to emerge again. These examples of teachers and neighbors working together shows us a sliver of what is possible when we activate our untapped collective power.

19

Love and live with abundance

Love big

I'm a woman living alone in New York at a very harrowing time. Maybe that should make me feel lonely, but the truth is that this whole experience has allowed me to embrace all the love in my life in all its different forms.

Through this experience, I received the love of friends who would provide a listening ear or drop off that extra batch of food at my door without being asked. I experienced the generosity of co-workers who reassured me that they would handle things while I was away so that I could focus on my recovery. I experienced the love of my siblings who checked in on me frequently and kept things light-hearted even when they must have been very worried about me. I felt the love of my 8-year-old niece who, upon finding out that I had the coronavirus, sent me a get-well note with 11 well-picked emojis! I felt appreciation for my mother, who is so strong and resilient that just learning from her example gave me strength in my own battle. I experienced the love of my father, who called me one day telling me that he has been waking up every day at four in the morning unable to sleep. He didn't have to say the words, but I said, "I got it, Dad. I love you too, and I'll be okay." I also experienced the love of strangers who reached out to me with their own stories of struggle and triumph and helped me get present to our shared humanity.

In the end, all it comes down to is love. A mental note to myself and to all of you: STOP being stingy! If you feel love, express it. And do it now! What have you got to lose? Love with abundance. It's not like it's running out of stock!

And accept love with abundance as well. Over the past few months, time slowed down for me, and I had nothing to do but just *be with* all the warmth I was receiving from so many people around the world. It was overwhelming at times. But when I finally let it really sink in, it was the most profoundly moving experience of my life. Now I know I have the capacity to notice the love that exists in my life, not just when I'm having a near-death experience but in all my everyday moments.

I hope you too begin to cultivate this capacity because I can tell you from first-hand experience that there is nothing more beautiful than allowing yourself to love and be loved. It's simple, really. But if that's all I take away from this journey, it will all have been worth it.

Live big

Turning points can be challenging, but they can also help us build resilience, rediscover the beauty in everyday things, connect with one another, awaken to what's possible, and activate our collective spirit.

And all this can be cultivated if we're willing to start with ourselves. Each of us has enormous power within us, more than we even know! I believe that if enough of us do this inner work to transform our-selves, something will absolutely transform in the world around us. When we each feel strong, safe, loved, and free to express our deepest selves, we cre-ate space for others around us to be this way as well.

Imagine if by expanding our inner selves, we each generated just a little more love in the immedi-ate spaces around us—with our families, co-workers, and communities, or even with cashiers at our neigh-borhood stores or the people we pass by on our daily commutes to work. Imagine what would be possible if each of us had a ripple effect on the ten people with whom we interact the most.

And if enough of us take this on in our own cir-cles, pretty soon we will activate a tipping point where whole systems around us start to transform.

Let's be brave! Let's allow ourselves to lean on others. Let's grow through our struggles. Let's sit still long enough to know ourselves. Let's express our love with fervor. Let's allow ourselves to be deeply moved by the beauty of simple things in life. Let's be com-passionate even when it's challenging. Let's acknowl-edge that each of us has something special to con-tribute to the world. Let's take more risks in sharing ourselves with others. Let's stand for a world where every living being is seen and heard.

Let's be brave now, and in doing so, inspire all those around us to be brave too!

It only takes one person to set a ripple effect in motion. So why not be the one?

Afterword

I started the year on top of the world (literally!) overlooking the gorgeous sapphire sea from a beautiful mountain range in Koh Samui, Thailand. A few months later, I was severely ill and fighting for my life. All the wishes I had made for the year while standing on top of that mountain vanished.

But as 2020 draws to a close, I'm surprisingly grateful for everything that's happened. It was the most difficult year of my life, and yet I'm ending it feeling more alive than ever before. While I have not recovered my full health, it has improved significantly over these past months, and I am grateful for that.

As I look ahead to the New Year, I choose to take all the lessons from this year with me. For my health, I wish for the strength to accept whatever comes my way. In my personal life, I wish to be fully present in precious moments with loved ones even when the world speeds up again. With my work, I'm committed now, more than ever, to reimagine education so that all children have the opportunity to discover the light within them and express themselves freely in the world.

My hope for you is that, no matter what life throws at you, you now have a few more tools to get unstuck, and to unlock your greatest self. Even if just one thing resonated with you from this book, I hope you try it on in your own life and see what you discover.

What a beautiful world it will be if we all choose to be BRAVE NOW. Good luck!

Acknowledgements

Writing this book gave me a sense of purpose amidst a challenging year. I poured away at these pages on many sleepless nights and weekends. I'll admit that, on certain days when the pain and fatigue got especially intense, I considered giving up on this project.

What kept me going were the tens of thousands of people out there who, just like me, have been battling this virus and its after-effects. My good wishes go out to everyone in the COVID-19 online support communities, with special gratitude to those of you who (although you may not even know it) brought me light on dark days.

I am also deeply grateful for the support of many incredible people in my life.

To my family, thank you for always being there for me. Mom, your strength and unconditional love are the greatest gifts. Radhika, I'm so lucky to have a warm and caring sister like you. Rajen, your high-spirited energy inspires me, as do our honest conversations about life. Dad, I know you are there for me if I ever need you.

To my friends who are like family: Sakshi, I can always count on you, and this year was no exception. I'm grateful for our eternal friendship and the light that you are in my life. Wendy, your unwavering support and genuine care were lifelines for me through all the chaos. Words can't express how much I appreciate you. Aaron, I'll never forget how you showed up for me in the middle of the night and in the days thereafter. Katherine, my return to work was a lot less scary because you held me with such compassion. Sid, your empathy and gentle encouragement kept me moving forward one baby step at a time. Erin, your resilient spirit is always an inspiration. Anubha and Vicky, I loved the laughter we shared throughout this crazy year. Shruti, I am grateful to you for helping me find the right care and also for your incredibly caring nature.

To Gary Williams, Sarah Barbour, Alejandro Martin, and the SPS community, I appreciate your positive encouragement and guidance as I navigated new territory.

And finally, to all the wise guides in my life: the many friends, coaches, and colleagues who have helped me grow; fellow writers who have expanded my horizons with ancient and new wisdom; my nieces and nephews who remind me of the wonderful realms of play and imagination; and the memorable strangers who have altered my life without even knowing it – thank you all for being my teachers.

I feel lucky to have so much love, support and wisdom in my life.

Notes

1   Radha Ruparell. "What No One Tells You About Having COVID-19", Medium (blog), April 23, 2020, https://medium.com/@radharuparell/what-no-one-tells-you-about-having-covid-19-97860a94eae

2   Jalāl al-Dīn Rūmī, Maulana, The Essential Rumi, translated by Coleman Barks. San Francisco: Harper, 1995.

3   "Werner Erhard – What's So" No Mind's Land (blog), August 26, 2019 https://nomindsland.blogspot.com/2019/08/werner-erhard-whats-so.html

4   Frankl, Viktor E. (Viktor Emil), 1905-1997. Man's Search for Meaning; an Introduction to Logotherapy. Boston: Beacon Press, 1962.

5   Larry Pearson. "Beyond the Vicious Circle", Landmark Insights,   https://landmarkinsights.com/2018/07/beyond-the-vicious-circle/

6   Seligman, M. E., Steen, T. A., Park, N., & Peterson, C. (2005). Positive psychology progress: empirical validation of interventions. The American psychologist, 60(5), 410–421. https://doi.org/10.1037/0003-066X.60.5.410

7   Kyeong, S., Kim, J., Kim, D. et al. (2017). Effects of gratitude meditation on neural network functional connectivity and brain-heart coupling. Scientific Reports, 7, 5058.

8   Aknin, L. B., Hamlin, J. K., Dunn, E. W. (2012). Giving leads to happiness in young children. PLoS ONE, 7(6), e39211.

Made in the USA
Monee, IL
03 June 2021

70076369R00142